JUST SAY KNOW

JUST SAY KNOW

Talking with Kids about Drugs and Alcohol

CYNTHIA KUHN, PH.D.,
SCOTT SWARTZWELDER, PH.D.,
AND
WILKIE WILSON, PH.D.

W. W. Norton & Company
New York   London

To Our Families

Photographs following page 64 reproduced courtesy of the Drug Enforcement Agency,
U.S. Department of Justice, Arlington, Virginia 22202.

Adolescent brain reproduced with permission from E. R. Sowell, P. M. Thompson, C. J.
Holmes, T. L. Jernigan, and A. W. Toga. "In Vivo Evidence for Post-Adolescent Brain
Maturation in Frontal and Striatal Regions," *Nature Neuroscience* 2 (10) 1999, 859.

For information about permission to reproduce selections from this book, write to
Permissions, W. W. Norton & Company, Inc., 500 Fifth Avenue, New York, NY 10110

The text of this book is composed in Berkeley Book
with display set in Impact and Futura Light.
Composition by Gina Webster.
Manufacturing by Courier Westford
Book design by Dana Sloan
Production manager: Julia Druskin

Library of Congress Cataloging-in-Publication Data

Kuhn, Cynthia.
Just say know : talking with kids about drugs and alcohol / Cynthia Kuhn, Scott Swartzwelder,
and Wilkie Wilson.
p.   cm.
Includes index.
ISBN 0-393-32258-0 (pbk.)
1. Children—Drug use—Prevention. 2. Children—Alcohol use—Prevention. 3. Drug abuse—
Prevention. 4. Alcoholism—Prevention. 5. Parenting. I. Title: Talking with kids about
drugs and alcohol. II. Swartzwelder, Scott. III. Wilson, Wilkie. IV. Title.
HV5824.C45 K84 2002
649'.4—dc21

2001044703

W. W. Norton & Company, Inc., 500 Fifth Avenue, New York, N.Y. 10110
www.wwnorton.com

W. W. Norton & Company, Ltd., Castle House, 75/76 Wells Street, London WIT 3QT

1 2 3 4 5 6 7 8 9 0

CONTENTS

JUST SAY KNOW

INTRODUCTION

This book is about hope. It is about how you can guide your children to develop a healthy respect for their brains and the rest of their bodies, how you can lead them to understand the importance of developing this respect, and how you can help them avoid the pitfalls of drugs.

The authors are parents and scientists. As parents, one of us has been through this phase and learned a lot, another is in the throes of it, and a third is beginning to face it. We know the fear of the phone call in the night. We know how stressful life can be as children grow from small frail bodies to beings with the bodies of adults but with brains still in transition between childhood and adulthood. We know that children have access to a large number of drugs (a larger number, more widely available than ever before) that will keep them up, take them down, or just make them feel better for a little while. Yet despite what you read, despite the scare stories the media hurl at you, we have every reason to believe that children can be safe and healthy.

As scientists, we lead research laboratories that are dedicated to understanding how the brain works and how chemicals change it. We want to help you understand how complicated and special our brains are—how they learn the strangest things, how they adapt to their environment. We also want to help you understand how precious the brains of children are.

The brains of children are so geared for learning that they absorb, like a sponge, everything around them, making maps of the world that will be with them for all of their lives. The messages adults give their children literally stay with them for life, encoded in the cells and chemicals of their brains. The younger they are, the more connections are being made and are yet to be made, so experiences, lessons, and behaviors learned early are those that are most fully incorporated into everything learned later. Thus, we believe the most effective education about drugs starts early.

On the other hand, it is never too late to start. Despite what kids may say, they think a lot about the issue of substance abuse. A recent poll showed that drug and alcohol use was the greatest concern among American teenagers. The teenager years are a time of natural curiosity, enormous anxiety, and incredible pressure to conform. In our experience, kids are anxious to talk about this subject under two conditions. First, they want to be taken seriously. They want their feelings of anxiety and stress recognized and accepted. They want to know that their parents have some idea what it is like to be in their shoes.

Second, they want to be told the truth about drugs. This is where most drug education fails miserably. In an attempt to scare kids into avoiding illicit drug use, many parents and educators stress the worst possible outcome from the use of a particular drug and frankly ignore the momentary positive feelings that the drug produces. But the human brain is complicated, and the various drugs that people use differ widely in their effects on the brain. These complex factors make talking about drugs much less simple than most people think it is.

Part of the problem parents have with learning about drugs is that not a lot of accessible information about drugs is available for parents to read. Very often, kids gain a lot more information from the street than their parents. Even if much of what the kids hear is wrong, there's just enough truth to hook them. The parents fall back on the "just say no" approach because they either cannot or will not become sufficiently informed to have a meaningful conversation. If "just say no" worked, that would be fine. It doesn't.

Kids are naturally curious, and as teenagers they are in a lot of emotional pain. They are also risk takers. Like it or not, kids have access to drugs that, for a short while, can entertain them, wake them up, put them to sleep, or just ease the pain. In Western society we live with the potent combination of automobiles, lots of free time, intense media stimulation, and the availability of a wide variety of drugs to change our mental state. This situation is unprecedented in human history, and dealing with it will take more than a slogan and a one-time admonition to "stay away from those drugs."

We wrote this book to give people enough information to educate themselves effectively and thus speak knowledgeably with children about drugs. We begin with a chapter that discusses communication with kids from the early years through adolescence. If parents can begin to develop trust between themselves and their children early on, most of the battle is won. Part of developing that trust is learning how to tell children what they need to know, without telling them more than they need. Early in life, children don't need to hear about intravenous drug injections and the diseases associated with that type of drug use. They need to hear how their brains contain the very essence of who they are and how they should nourish their brains with good food and healthy habits. Later in life, adolescents need to hear the same message, but with more detailed information along with it.

The second chapter teaches parents some very basic information about how drugs interact with the body. It describes the various ways that drugs can enter the body, how they move into the brain, and how the body gets rid of them. It also describes in general the ways in which drugs can harm the body. It outlines the process of addiction and how people become dependent on drugs. Finally, it describes the health risks associated with the drug-oriented lifestyle, many of which most people do not know.

Chapter 3—one of the most important—is a reminder of the legal issues that always surround drug use. We are not lawyers, and this is not official legal advice. But it is very important that parents and kids understand the legal ramifications of becoming involved with drugs. One of the most important concepts for a child to understand is how easy it is to get caught in a legal nightmare, even if that child is relatively innocent. The laws have become so strict and far-reaching that the slightest infraction can result in terrible penalties, especially now that children can be tried as adults. Kids, who are always the first to say "That's not fair!," need to understand that even getting them "fair" treatment can generate legal bills that will bankrupt most families.

After these introductions, the following chapters deal with individual classes of drugs. These range from the mildest, caffeine, to the very addictive, cocaine. There are chapters for alcohol, stimulants, depressants, hallucinogens, Ecstasy, and several others. For each drug class, there is a summary of the short-term and long-term risks of using the drugs, a description of how they make a person feel, and some important points to make when talking to kids about their use. These chapters are designed to give parents the information they need, along with some guidance, without overburdening them with great detail. We also have provided pictures of many commonly used drugs.

We hope that the information in this book helps lots of kids and parents move toward a trusting relationship that allows both the parents and the children to talk effectively to one another. The former head of the Office of National Drug Policy, General

Barry McCaffrey, said that drug education has to happen at the kitchen table. He's right. No one can educate a child as well as his or her parents. In fact, almost all of this book can be helpful in guiding and helping kids who are already having drug problems. It is written to help adults understand how the brain works and how drugs affect it, what addiction is and is not, and how to communicate effectively with kids.

1. COMMUNICATION IS KEY

Start Early

There is no question that good drug education begins in the home and quickly extends into the many other places that a child spends time. It also begins early in the life of a child. Long before having a conversation about the health risks of drinking alcohol or using other drugs, children can be taught important lessons about how the body works and the ways it can be vulnerable to the effects of chemicals. If a child learns to respect and take care of his body, he'll be more likely to think carefully later in life about the kinds of foods, medicines, and drugs he puts into it.

These lessons can be taught from an early age. Simply taking the time to explain in basic terms how a child's body works, when the opportunities arise, is a great start. We think of these as "teachable moments." For example, when a two year old has a stomachache it's nice to reassure him that he'll feel better soon. It's also easy to explain that some of the things we can eat are not so good for the stomach and can cause a stomachache. This kind of simple explanation can help a child to begin thinking about how his body works and to understand that not everything that we can put into our bodies is good for us.

Backyard scrapes can also provide teachable moments. As you clean up a child's cut she might be curious or fearful about seeing blood on her knee. This could be an opportunity to explain that blood isn't a scary or bad thing, but in fact flows throughout the entire body and carries energy from the foods we eat to the brain so we can think, to the muscles so we can move and play, and to the bones and joints so we can grow. You might be surprised at the interest and questions you get in response to explanations like these. But you don't have to be a physiologist or physician to answer them. Simply telling what you know sends the important message that you care about the child's body and health and that the body is not a mysterious cavern but a wondrous collection of parts that make sense and make us who we are.

Minor infections are great teaching opportunities too. When a child has an ear infection and is on a course of antibiotics, this is an opportunity to introduce several important ideas. First, there is a difference between a drug and a food. A drug is taken for a specific reason—to get rid of the germs that are making him sick—and only for the time that it's necessary. Second, drugs should only be taken after consulting with a doctor, because the doctor has taken a long time to learn what's good for him and when. If the child is curious about how a medicine that he swallows can help his ear to feel better, you have an opportunity to explain how the things we eat and drink are distributed by the blood to everywhere in the body.

You don't have to force these kinds of issues into your dialogue. Casual mention of any of these points can make an impression. Children often take in new information silently and then follow up later with a question when they've had time to digest it. We've found a parallel in discussions with our kids about sex. They seem to ask for only as much information as they need or can interpret at the time. More sophisticated questions—and more detailed conversation—come later. The point is that a casual comment with a little information can plant a seed that may evolve into a series of important conversations later. The other benefit is that your mentioning the issue gives the child permission to think about it—and, most important, to ask you about it later.

This is perhaps the single most important goal—to have children become comfortable talking with you about "difficult" topics, such as drugs, sex, and relationships. If you plant the seeds for that kind of trust early by being calm, open, and available, you've set the stage for great communication down the road.

Listen Carefully and Know What You're Talking About

As children get older, their questions get harder to answer. This is good because it provides more opportunity for detailed discussion, but it presents some challenges too. The best way to prepare for this is to become informed about drugs and to learn to listen carefully. Too many conversations about drugs never happen because the adult feels uncomfortable or "unqualified" to carry it off. The more you know, the less that can take you by surprise and the more opportunities you'll find to initiate conversations about drugs . . . "Did you see that newspaper article about low doses of alcohol protecting against heart disease?" . . . "I saw a TV show the other night about a drug called Ecstasy—seems like pretty dangerous stuff." Children and adolescents face a dizzying array of information, and much of it is rather poor. They may think they've gotten the facts on a drug because they've read something on an internet site or in a magazine, but these sources are notoriously unreliable. If you are aware of the basic scientific facts, you'll be in a great position to challenge misinformation and myths calmly.

Being a good listener is also a powerful way to get your points across. When a child or teen can tell that you are really listening, it communicates not only that you care, but also that you understand what they are saying. Both are critical. Thus it's important to let the child say all she has to say about the issue. Even if some of what she says frightens or angers you, it's important to let her have her say. It's also okay to let her know how you feel about what she thinks, but remember that she may also feel frightened or angry about the topic and may be relying on you to remain calm and supportive. For all their apparent independence and rebellion, teens are still kids deep down and look to adults for direction and encouragement. So your job is to strike a balance between using your power and influence over their lives and providing support and encouragement. Much of this boils down to how you *manage your authority*.

There is a very big difference between being *authoritative* and being *authoritarian*. An authoritarian response is one that falls back on power without considering much else . . . "because I said so!" Once a conversation with a teen becomes a power struggle, nobody wins. An authoritative response is much different. It relies much more on knowledge than power. The power is a backdrop to the conversation (kids know this without having to be told), but it is not in the forefront. In an authoritative stance you listen to be sure that your responses are addressing the right issues. Then you use your knowledge and experience to lay out a reasoned viewpoint and response. This does not mean that you don't wield your authority, but rather that you use it optimally, in ways that engage, rather than alienate, the child you're talking with.

What do you say, and when? There are no clear-cut prescriptions. To a great degree, you must rely on your own knowledge of the child with whom you are dealing. Research shows that the middle school years are when kids really learn about drugs. This makes sense because their mental abilities and their social environments are changing. They are becoming more independent and learning to question authority. In the following chapters of this book, we've made a number of suggestions about what to say to kids. Many of these suggestions are appropriate for teens because it is during the teen years that you are most likely to have direct conversations about drugs. But as we've emphasized above, younger kids can also learn to appreciate their bodies and how to keep them healthy. Of course, some young kids will come to you with specific questions about drugs—after seeing a reference in the media, hearing a story in the playground, or going through an elementary school drug education program. In these instances we recommend answering the questions directly and listening to determine how much the child really wants to know. Don't try to force too much information on a young child. If you have good communication with him, he'll ask for more when he's ready. In summary, talk with young kids about the general ideas of good health and how the brain and the rest of the body work, and talk more specifically about drugs and drug effects with teens and college students.

Empower Kids to Make Their Own Decisions

The communication strategies we described above give a child both the permission and the information necessary to make healthy decisions. The next challenge is to trust and monitor that process. Sooner or later children grow up and begin to think for themselves no matter what we do. This means that, as parents or mentors, we have only a limited time to have a positive influence. It's important to use that time well.

We have to provide more than just scientific facts, love, and support. It's also important to let kids know that they can resist pressure from peers and the media to use drugs and take other risks. All children will experience these pressures—it's just not possible to insulate them completely—so we have to let them know that the decisions are theirs. We can be available to help, but there will be many times that they won't come to us and we have to feel comfortable that we have equipped them as best we can.

Sometimes all it takes to empower a child to resist pressures is the knowledge that not all people use or even try drugs. Alcohol abuse by college students is a good example. During the past several years so much attention has been given to so-called binge drinking on college campuses that many incoming freshmen assume that nearly every student drinks excessively. The truth is that, although about 20 percent of college students engage in heavy drinking, a comparable percentage are total abstainers, and the rest fall into the middle range, which represents moderate drinking. When provided with this information, many young students are relieved to know that they do not have to engage in heavy drinking to fit in at college. There are some excellent ongoing surveys that track the drug use patterns of children and teens. Most of the media attention to these surveys focuses on the trends—how many more kids are using now than five years ago, etc.

Establish Clear Family Rules and Be Consistent

It is not hard to understand that young children are comforted by stability and consistency. They might not always like the rules themselves, but they appreciate and need the clarity. When parents' expectations and reactions are clear and consistent, children know where they stand. Then when they encounter the less predictable world outside the family, they are able to engage it with confidence.

If you're a parent and have a partner in the home, the two of you should talk first about what the family rules should be. It's important that the adults involved be on the same page. If you're alone, take some time to think through what the rules of your household should be. Ask for advice. What are your goals? If you are a teacher, friend, mentor, minister, or clinician who is dealing with a family, remember that the rules you might put in place in your own home are not necessarily what's best for the other family. If you're asked for advice, listen carefully to what the family tells you about how they live and what they think is important. That way, you can be a more objective and effective advisor.

In that spirit, we are not going to endorse any specific family rules. But we do suggest a "hands-on" rather than a "hands-off" approach. In general, the more involved parents or caretakers are with children's lives, the less likely the children are to get into trouble with drugs, and the more likely they are to report having meaningful relationships with their parents.

But where do you start? One place might be to take a look at what kinds of rules have proven useful for others. A recent study of about a thousand U.S. teens by the National Center on Addiction and Substance Abuse looked at twelve family actions and asked if incorporating them into the family rules affected the kids' family relationships or likelihood of using drugs. They asked whether parents:

- Monitor what their teens watch on TV
- Monitor what their teens do on the internet
- Put restrictions on the CDs they buy
- Know where their teens are after school and on weekends
- Are told the truth by their teens about where they are going
- Are "very aware" of their teens' academic performance
- Impose a curfew
- Make clear they would be "extremely upset" if their teen used pot
- Eat dinner with their teens six or seven nights a week

- Turn off the TV during dinner
- Assign their teens regular chores
- Have an adult present when the teens return home from school

These actions are all indicators of a hands-on approach to raising teens. The researchers considered a family to be hands-on if the parents consistently incorporate ten or more of these rules in family life. In hands-on families, 47 percent of teens reported having an "excellent" relationship with their fathers and 57 percent with their mothers. Only 13 and 24 percent of kids from hands-off families reported excellent relationships with their fathers and mothers, respectively. That's a huge difference! Being hands-on has an extremely powerful positive effect on family relationships, which makes sense. If you know where your kids are after school and eat with them six or seven nights a week, you are simply going to know each other better. Good things usually grow from there. Kids from the hands-on families were also at lower risk for smoking, drinking, and using illegal drugs.

Adults Are Role Models for Drug Use—Do It Right!

Children often look to adults for guidance without directly asking for it—sometimes they just watch and copy. Educators and psychologists call this process "modeling" because kids tend to model much of their own behavior on what they see adults doing. It can be frightening to look at our behavior and see things that we hope children won't copy. But modeling is also rife with opportunities for teaching without saying a word.

If children see you making careful decisions about your own health and drug use, they will learn to take a careful approach to such decisions as well. One of the most important things a child can see you do is ask questions as part of a decision-making process about what you put into your body. Nobody knows all there is to know about medicines, dietary supplements, vitamins, and over-the-counter remedies. When your children see you reading an information label and discussing it with your doctor, pharmacist, spouse, or friend, they learn that it's okay to admit not knowing about drugs and to ask questions and discuss options.

This also sends the message that the information needed to make healthy decisions is available. Good sources of information exist, and children should know that they are out there and accessible. On the other hand, there is a lot of bad information available too—particularly on the internet, where there's essentially zero quality control. So it's also important to show that you consider your information sources carefully.

Modeling raises two other important issues: what to tell children about your own recreational drug experiences, and why it's seen as okay for adults to use certain drugs that are restricted for children and adolescents. Many of today's parents, educators, and counselors have had some experience with recreational drugs, and that experience can be useful in communicating with children whether or not you choose to disclose the experiences specifically. But should you tell a teen about your own drug experiences?

No single answer will work for everyone. Clearly, in the eyes of some drug treatment therapists and peer counselors, one's revelations about previous drug use can be part of the treatment process. This is a clinical issue that is out of our range in this book. But what about others—parents, teachers, ministers, guidance counselors? Here you have to weigh some important pros and cons. The most compelling reason to avoid sharing your own drug history is that it conveys a kind of permission: "You did it, so what's the big deal?" The arguments that "things were different then" or "the drugs were less potent in those days" just don't hold water.

On the other hand, some would argue that coming clean about your own casual drug use can promote a sense of honest communication between you and a teen. Maybe so. But remember that kids and adults don't always interpret things in the same way. What you might experience as an honest, open conversation could be confusing or even frightening to a teen. Again, this is an individual decision that must be taken very seriously. On balance, we urge caution when it comes to revealing your own drug experiences.

Whether or not you choose to reveal your personal use, it is very important to consider a related issue: Why it is acceptable for adults to do some things that kids should not do? Alcohol and nicotine are legal for adults but not for kids. Are there good reasons for this, or is it just an authoritarian stance? We think there are good reasons, and they provide a great opportunity to teach some simple but critical things about the brain. It is now clear that the adolescent (and young adult) brain is still in a period of rapid developmental change. This fact conveys both great opportunity and great risk. Put simply, the adolescent and young adult brain has not finished growing, and the growth that is yet to happen is essential to a person's ability to function socially and cognitively in adulthood. Adolescence is a dangerous time to be messing around with brain circuitry, when it is still being sculpted into its final adult form.

Adults' Brains and Children's Brains Are Different

The fact that adults' brains and children's brains are different has probably been obvious to teens and parents for centuries, but now it is known just how big the difference really is. Not so long ago (when we were in training as young neuroscientists), we were taught that all of the important brain development was completed fairly early in childhood. But now it is understood that brain development proceeds *at least* into a person's early twenties. Many of the people that we have spoken with have found this new scientific information to be one of the most effective tools for communicating with children about drugs.

The part of the brain that appears to undergo the most developmental change during adolescence is a large region just behind the forehead called the *frontal lobes*. The most recent medical imaging studies are showing this finding, as illustrated in the figure in the insert following page 64. The frontal lobes are perhaps the region most responsible for giving us the capacity to process highly challenging kinds of information and plan our lives in an orderly and effective way. Because these frontal lobe functions have such a powerful effect on organizing our other mental functions, they have come to be called "executive functions." The role the frontal lobes play in organizing the functions of other brain regions is viewed like the role of an executive in a corporation—they coordinate and direct others' actions toward specific complex goals. When the frontal lobes are damaged or become diseased, a person suffers deficits in her ability to plan and execute goals, learn complex kinds of information, and solve problems. She may also have difficulty with self-control and fail to appreciate the implications of her own behavior.

Researchers are just beginning to investigate the unique effects that drugs have on the developing brain, but we already know that the effects of alcohol can be quite different depending on a person's age (see the Alcohol chapter for more on this), and the same may be true for other drugs. The really scary question is whether exposing the brain to certain drugs during development can change the way the brain develops—possibly altering brain function for life. We have known for decades that exposure to alcohol and other chemicals during prenatal brain development can damage the brain. Now we have to consider the possibility that later exposures can do so as well.

Spotting and Responding to a Problem

There is no clear-cut formula for recognizing when a kid begins to get into trouble with drugs. Sometimes a parent, teacher, or coach just has a hunch that something is wrong. Sometimes there are clearer warning signs. It's important to pay attention to your hunches, but not to overreact. Likewise, some of the typical warning signs could be present without any drug use at all, so good judgment and a calm, measured approach is always best. Here are some signs that should get your attention.

Changes in Behavior or Attitude

- An abrupt drop in grades or school activities
- Decreased involvement or talkativeness at home
- An abrupt change in friends
- Loss of motivation, particularly for previously favorite activities
- Increased need for money
- Secretiveness, irritability, lying
- Problems with learning, memory, attention

Physical Changes

- Loss of energy
- Changes in appetite or weight
- Changes in speech patterns—slurring, slowing, rapid, or pressured speech
- Dilated pupils, consistently red eyes

While these signs can be helpful as first indicators of trouble, remember that any of them can occur for reasons other than drug use. Everybody responds a little differently to stress, life changes, and drug effects, so knowing a child well makes it a lot easier to notice changes that may indicate a problem. If you've had the opportunity to build a consistent, communicative relationship, then you are more likely to notice such changes. For example, a kid who is generally talkative within the family or at school may begin to withdraw from those relationships. You're not going to notice this if you haven't been talking with her regularly. If you do notice her backing off or becoming more quiet, though, it's important not to jump to conclusions. There are lots of reasons that kids, particularly teens, may "go quiet" for periods of time. Remember, many physical and social changes are taking place as kids grow. You can approach her in a calm and caring way, note that you've observed a change, and ask if there is anything she wants to talk about or if there's any way for you to help. Even if she turns down the offer, just coming to her may provide a needed feeling of safety and support.

If you remain concerned about a possible problem, it's important to keep your eyes and ears open while avoiding unnecessary confrontation and the temptation to become a detective always looking for "evidence." Kids may discover you're spying on them and react by becoming even more secretive and distrustful. That's not to say you should take a hands-off approach—just the opposite. This is the time to be as involved as possible, but you must combine your concerned observation of her behavior with the consistent message that you remain "on her side" no matter what. This is a difficult balance, and there is no set prescription for how to carry it off. Perhaps an example from one of us can provide a framework for thinking about your own situation.

One day when Scott's daughter was thirteen, he delivered a basket of clean laundry to her bedroom. When she came home and discovered it, she came to him, perturbed, and asked that he not go back into her room while she was not there. Scott saw the opportunity to define some rules and do some relationship building. She explained that she wanted her room to be a private place for her and that the thought of someone going in and out in her absence made her feel uncomfortable. Scott suppressed the urge to remind her of who paid the mortgage and, instead, told her that he completely appreciated her urge for privacy and that he felt the same way about his private space. But as her parent, he explained, he had responsibilities for her welfare that made his respect for her privacy just a little complicated. He felt stuck on how to explain the conflict between respect for her privacy and his responsibility to keep her safe until an example came to mind. He reminded her of his clinical work. "You know that when I see patients at the hospital, I am required to keep secret what they tell me. I have to respect their privacy (just as I do yours). Otherwise they won't be able to tell me the things that I need to know in order to help them." She understood both the clinical importance of trust and the ethical obligation of clinician-patient confidentiality. Scott went on— "But I always have to tell my patients at the very beginning of treatment that if I come to believe that they are a danger to themselves or others, I must tell the proper people in order to keep them safe." She understood. "So, how about we have the same agreement about your room? I trust you, and I think you make good decisions. So, I'll stay out of your room as long as I am confident that you are taking good care of yourself and aren't doing anything to put yourself in danger." That is still the standing arrangement between them. Both of them got most of what they wanted. Scott's daughter got the assurance of privacy in her room, while Scott retained the option to go in if he really became concerned about her. Most important, they maintained a relationship based on mutual trust and made an important agreement based on that trust.

What if you discover a problem? The first thing to remember is that you will be most effective if you act promptly and decisively, *but not alone*! Drug use problems are complex and require professional attention—preferably from a team of clinicians including both medical and behavioral experts. If you live near a major medical center there is probably a drug treatment clinic available, and many of these have specific clinics devoted to adolescents. Your family doctor or school counselor may be able to help find the right clinic for treatment. There also may be a drug hot line listed in the phone book that can put you in touch with someone who can help you manage your own immediate feelings as well as set up a treatment strategy.

If you're not in a place where you can take advantage of a treatment team, it's important to know that different professionals will likely take different approaches to a kid with drug problems. A medical professional (physician, nurse, or physician's assistant) will probably think first about the physical side of the problem and want to make sure that there is no acute medical crisis. This is always a good place to start. Once it's determined that no medical problem exists, though, a medical professional is more likely to try to refer you to someone with more of a behavioral treatment orientation, such as a psychiatrist, psychologist, or social worker. These professionals often have overlapping skills and may take very different approaches to the problem. Psychiatrists are medical doctors who are specifically trained to use medicines to help with problems of thinking and behavior. Some will also include psychotherapy. So it's important to discuss with a psychiatrist whether she will try to use medicines to help, or if she'll take more of a psychotherapeutic (i.e., talking) approach. Clinical psychologists are licensed clinicians who are specifically trained to use psychotherapy and other behavioral techniques to change behavior, thinking, and feelings. They do not prescribe medications, but they may "prescribe" specific kinds of behavioral exercises or homework to help a person break the behavior patterns that may be leading to the drug use. Social workers are also not medical professionals and do not prescribe medications, but they may use psychotherapy and behavioral techniques in an effort to break the cycle of drug use. Social workers and psychologists are often interested in working with the family as well as the patient. The underlying theory is that drug problems do not happen in isolation and that an understanding of how the family works can be of great help.

No matter what kind of treatment professional you engage, two things are critical—the person must be licensed and must have experience dealing with drug problems. There are state licensing boards for physicians, psychologists, and social workers, as well as for drug counselors. Be sure that the person you are dealing with is qualified.

2. DRUG BASICS

We are a drug-taking culture. We take nutritional supplements, antibiotics to cure infections, drugs to cure disease, and drugs to mildly stimulate or relax us. We treat serious disease like asthma, high blood pressure, and cancer. We take vitamins and eat herb- and vitamin-fortified foods. These habits are often helpful and have led to one of the healthiest populations in the world. However, a few drugs present such appeal that occasional use leads some people to compulsive, health-damaging cycles of drug seeking and taking.

On the one hand, the advertising industry exhorts us through every available medium—radio, TV, and newspaper and magazines—to use drugs and supplements. We need to be careful to verify claims that are made in ads. On the other hand, many people have a growing concern about drugs and superstitiously avoid even drugs needed to treat disease. Some of these same people use herbal remedies of unknown composition or effectiveness instead—hardly an improvement.

The first step in talking to kids about drugs is to talk about what drugs are and to distinguish between drugs that treat disease and drugs that are health-damaging and addictive. The aim of this chapter is to help you understand drugs in general and lead you to look at your own attitudes about drug taking.

THE MOST IMPORTANT THINGS TO KNOW ABOUT DRUGS

1. What Is a Drug?

A drug is any substance that a person puts in his or her body with the intention of changing how it works. The physical properties (plant or chemical), cost, reason (treatment of disease or recreation), or source (prescription or food supplement) don't change whether or not a substance is considered to be a drug. Here is a short list of substances that are considered drugs, including some you might not have expected, with brief comments about general issues regarding drugs.

Nutritional Supplements: Vitamins, specific nutritional supplements such as amino acids, and many herbs are sold in health food stores and grocery stores. People take these as pills in addition to the vitamins and nutrients that they eat in their food. Although these substances are required by the body, it is possible to take too much of some of them. For example, although it is rare, taking too much vitamin A can make a person sick.

Nutritional Supplements in Foods: Vitamins are added to some foods (milk, bread, cereal) automatically. This practice has virtually eliminated vitamin deficiency diseases in the United States. The amounts provided are appropriate and provide a useful way to maintain optimal nutrition.

Herbal Drugs: Herbal medications are sold specifically as drugs in herbal form—as loose herbs, teas, or capsules. They are also appearing in fortified drinks and snacks. The problem with these preparations is that there is no control over the quality or quantity sold. Some, like ephedrine (ma huang), are effective but can cause problems if too much is taken. Others, like ginseng and gingko, are of unproven medical benefit. They probably do no harm, but their definite health benefits have not yet been proven.

Caffeine: Caffeine is a psychoactive drug (a drug that changes behavior by working in the brain) that is present in many beverages, including sodas, coffee, and tea, as well as in small quantities in chocolate. Caffeine is also present in over-the-counter preparations for headache, for staying awake, and for fat burning.

Alcoholic Beverages: Alcohol in beverage form that is ingested with a meal, like beer or wine, is an example of a psychoactive drug in common foods.

Nicotine: Nicotine is available in many forms. It is usually taken in cigarettes, cigars, snuff, or chewing tobacco. Nicotine chewing gum and nicotine patches are now widely used for smoking cessation.

Over-the-Counter Medications: Many drugs that formerly required a prescription now can be obtained without one. We can treat ourselves with pain-reducing drugs such as aspirin, and drugs to treat heartburn, stuffy nose, cough, yeast infection, and a host of other ailments. In most cases, these drugs are safe, which is why they can be purchased without a prescription. However, a person must always consider how they interact with each other, and with drugs from other categories being taken at the same time, as well as with certain foods such as grapefruit that affect the absorption of all drugs.

Prescription Medications: Drugs that can only be obtained by a prescription from a doctor are powerful and may have dangerous side effects. In addition to drugs used to treat physical illnesses, such as infections, there are many beneficial drugs that can be used to treat diseases of the mind, such as anxiety, depression, and schizophrenia. As with over-the-counter drugs, they can interact with drugs obtained from other sources, such as herbal remedies and drugs in foods.

"Recreational" Drugs: Recreational drugs are what most people refer to as "drugs." What they mean are the substances taken intentionally to change behavior. The usual list includes marijuana, cocaine, amphetamine, opiates such as heroin, and hallucinogens such as LSD and Ecstasy. All of these drugs affect the brain. Many are illegal because they have no valid medical use (LSD is an example). Others have valid medical uses, but normally should be given only by prescription (amphetamine, morphine). They are *not* all addictive, nor are they all *narcotics* (a commonly misused term). Narcotics are drugs such as heroin or codeine that induce a state of drugged sleep.

Drugs People Don't Think of as Drugs: Frequently, when people are asked to list the drugs they take, they think only of their prescription medications and omit many other things, such as the sodas they drink at lunch (source of caffeine), cigarettes, birth control pills, herbal teas, or vitamin supplements.

Taking substances to affect our health is not uniquely human. Certain types of monkeys pick medicinal foods to eat when they are sick. For example, monkeys infested with parasites have been shown to eat the leaves of a particular kind of plant containing substances that kill parasites. When they are parasite-free, they don't touch these particular plants. Nobody understands how the monkeys know to medicate themselves this way.

Humans are not the only species to intoxicate themselves intentionally. The stimulating effect of caffeine supposedly was discovered by tribesmen who noticed how energetic their goats became when they ate particular berries. It is no accident that many of the behavior-changing drugs that we know, including nicotine, caffeine, cocaine, opiate-like drugs such as morphine and codeine, atropine, and many hallucinogens, are compounds made by plants. Why plants make these compounds remains a much-debated mystery. Are they encouraging animals to eat them to promote dispersal of their seeds? Or are they trying to discourage predation? It is probably some combination of both.

The bottom line is that people take drugs to change how their bodies work. This is useful and necessary for survival, and we shouldn't be superstitious about the dangers of drugs. However, we should also be careful shoppers and not give in to appeals to buy expensive remedies that don't work or to substitute unregulated "natural" herbal supplements that are unknown in potency or quality for medicines known to be safe and effective.

2. How Do Drugs Work?

Drugs must go where they are needed and then do what is wanted when they get there, without doing too much else. In this section, we discuss these two processes. The value of this information goes far beyond education about drug abuse. This is basic information that people need to understand in order to make intelligent decisions about their own bodies.

How do drugs get to where they are needed? Sometimes, it is possible to put drugs exactly where they need to be. This is the best possible situation. For example, we can treat the itchy rash that poison ivy causes by rubbing cream directly on the affected patch of skin. Besides treating skin disease, we can treat asthma by inhaling medicine, placing it directly in the respiratory tract where it is needed. We can treat some diseases of the eye by placing drops directly in the eye. In other cases, though, drugs must enter the bloodstream and be carried to where they are needed. This means that they must first get into the bloodstream, not always an easy task. It also means that, once there, they are free to go everywhere in the body. It is just not possible to send a drug specifically to the liver, for example, or to the pancreas. This is the major reason for drug side effects—we cannot restrict where drugs go once they enter the body.

The easiest way to get drugs into the bloodstream is by injecting them directly into the bloodstream (intravenously) or nearby (just under the skin or into the muscle). Some drugs must be given this way. For example, the insulin that diabetics use must be taken by injection because it is a large protein that would be broken down in the stomach. Although fast (and preferred by many addicts), injection routes can be dangerous because of the risk of overdose or infection. One of the biggest risks to heroin users today, besides death by overdose, is the transmission of the AIDS virus, HIV, through shared needles. In New York City, doctors estimate that 30 percent of addicts also have HIV from sharing needles for injection.

The other way to get drugs into the body quickly is to inhale them. This doesn't work for all drugs, but if they can be absorbed across the lungs, it is the next best thing to injecting them. This is why smoking cigarettes and crack cocaine works so well. The lungs provide a huge surface surrounded by blood vessels, so drugs can enter the circulation very quickly. Inhaling drugs intranasally (that is, snorting them) is a more restricted version of the same idea. In this case, drugs cross through the thin mucous membranes of the nose to enter the circulation. However, the average nose provides a lot less room than the average pair of lungs, and so it is not as effective a method.

The easiest way to take a drug is to swallow it. However, a swallowed drug must be absorbed through the lining of the digestive tract before it enters the bloodstream. A recent TV ad contrasting how antacids and a popular histamine-blocking drug work portrayed this situation pretty accurately—the his- tamine-blocking drug that decreases stomach acid must travel through the digestive tract, to the heart, and then get pumped back to the stomach to have its effect. For most drugs, how- ever, there is not a big hurry, and this safe and effective means works well.

What do drugs do when they get there? Drugs travel through the body until they find a molecule to which they can stick. You can envision the drug as a key, which eventually fits into a particular lock on a cell. The lock is called a receptor. Wherever the lock is located, the drug sticks, "unlocks" the lock, and changes what is going on in that cell. This is how drugs work and the reason for drug side effects.

The nose drops used to treat stuffy noses provide a great example. The active drug in nose drops sticks to receptors located on the blood vessels, causing the blood vessels to con- strict, which decreases the amount of blood in the nose and makes it less stuffy. When the drug is delivered directly into the nose, there is no problem: just the blood vessels in the nose are treated. However, this medicine also can be taken orally. When taken as pills or syrup, it travels throughout the whole body. These receptors are located on many blood vessels throughout the body, not just in the nose. Therefore, taking too much of this medicine can cause so much constriction of blood vessels that a person's blood pressure rises. This can be dangerous to people who already have high blood pressure and is a perfect example of how the useful effect of the drug cannot easily be separated from the cause of its side effects.

The nose drops we described above provide another example of why drugs have side effects. When you treat a stuffy nose, you are taking a normal system and making it abnormal. Your nose gets stuffy when you have a cold or allergies because a group of substances triggered by the immune response to an allergen or to a virus has caused fluid to gather there. We don't have any good way to turn off this process. So instead, we take a perfectly normal blood vessel receptor and stimulate it when it normally would not be stimulated. The birth control pill is another good example of taking a perfectly healthy body and changing it. This usually causes more problems than treating a disease. Treating a disease in some ways is easier. For example, when the thyroid gland fails to function, taking thyroid hormone can replace what is missing, thereby making an abnormal system normal again.

The bottom line about drugs and their receptors is that the reason they work on a particular system is not because they travel specifically to that system; drugs go everywhere. A drug that binds to a receptor in the liver affects how the liver works; if that same drug binds to a receptor on the blood vessels, it affects blood pressure. The good effects of drugs and their bad side effects generally result from the same actions, but in different places.

TV ads provide a great way to start this conversation with kids. Some ads are truthful, but some of them are not exactly accurate about how the drugs get to where they are needed in the body. Of course the ad claims that the product always gets to where it needs to be better and faster than the competition, and stays there longer, and causes fewer side effects. However, some of these wonderful qualities are mutually exclusive. For example, the drug that stays in the body for much longer might well have worse side effects than one that is eliminated quickly.

3. Why Do Drugs Stop Working?

Some drugs stop working if they are used continuously. The nose drops described above provide a good example. The drugs in nose drops are very effective during the first few uses. But most people notice that if they keep using them for days and days, they get less and less benefit from them. Eventually, some people start having a stuffy nose *unless* they use the nose drops. They can get trapped in a cycle of continuous use that is hard to break, because when they stop they experience the same stuffy nose that they were trying to treat in the first place.

This situation is typical tolerance. *Tolerance* is the state that exists when a drug stops working. What happens during tolerance is that the specific places where the "locks" for the nose drops occur gradually adapt to the presence of the nose drops. Pretty soon, they function normally only if the nose drops are present. *Dependence* is the flip side of tolerance: It describes the state in which a person's body functions normally only in the presence of the drug. The end stage described above, when the nose drop user has a stuffy nose unless he or she uses nose drops, is physical dependence. *Withdrawal* is what it feels like to be dependent. When the nose drop user stops using nose drops and has a terrible stuffy nose, he or she is going through decongestant withdrawal.

The headache that regular caffeine users get when they stop drinking caffeine is an example of dependence that might be familiar even to kids if they drink lots of caffeinated beverages. The "weekend headache" that regular office coffee drinkers can experience on Saturday morning away from the office is an example of a withdrawal effect caused by dependence on caffeine. Some children who are heavy soda drinkers have a Monday morning headache for the opposite reason—they don't get soda at school! This doesn't mean that a person is addicted to caffeine.

It has nothing to do with what caffeine does in the brain at all. We think it is caused by gradual changes in the blood vessels in the head, like the gradual changes that were described above for the nose drops.

Tolerance, dependence, and withdrawal do not occur just with illegal drugs, drugs of abuse, narcotics, or even psychoactive drugs. These are states that can occur after any drug is given for a long time. The gradual failure of antibiotics to work in some situations is another type of tolerance. In this case, the whole population of bacteria becomes tolerant in a special way. The affected individuals in the bacteria colony die, but individuals that are resistant to the drug survive and grow.

4. How Do Drugs Work in the Brain?

The way that drugs work in the brain is the same as in other systems: For drugs to affect how we feel or act, they must enter the nervous system and unlock the locks, or receptors, that are located there. Both events are important. There is a cellular barrier that keeps a lot of substances in the bloodstream out of the brain. All the drugs that we take to affect how we feel, including recreational drugs such as alcohol and drugs used to treat disease such as fluoxetine (Prozac), are able to cross this barrier.

Once a drug gets into the brain, it attaches to whatever receptor it sticks to. The basic process is no different from the nose drops causing blood vessels to constrict. The difference is that the cells in the brain—neurons—are involved in controlling every aspect of our behavior. This ranges from automatic functions (such as control of our breathing and heartbeat), voluntary movements, eating, drinking, and control of other important bodily functions, to complicated functions, such as emotions and memory. Receptors for drugs that act on the brain are almost never just in one part of the brain. The rarer they are, the fewer life functions are affected. The best drugs used to treat diseases are those that affect only a few neurons, so that the diseased condition can be treated without affecting other brain functions. However, most drugs affect many neurons. A drug like alcohol, which affects a receptor that exists throughout the brain, is capable of affecting almost every function of the brain.

5. What Is Addiction? What Drugs Are Addictive?

So if caffeine withdrawal headaches aren't addiction, what is addiction? *Addiction is the repeated, compulsive use of a substance that continues even though the addict is experiencing bad consequences.* The key to the definition is the loss of control over use. When someone is an addict, the process of taking the drug has control over his or her life. He doesn't do the things he used to do, but develops new friendships, often based on drug taking, and no longer has time for the normally rewarding activities he once enjoyed. Kids that we know have commented that when their friends get really involved in drugs, they aren't fun anymore, because all they do is hang out with other kids who use drugs.

According to this definition, someone who snorts cocaine once a month, and can take it or leave it, is not an addict. Fairly regular users of marijuana often make this argument. So why should you worry if your child defends his or her drug use because he or she has it under control? You should worry because occasional use of certain drugs can be so compelling that it develops into addictive patterns of use, and many factors influence who slides down this slippery slope.

The good news is that not many drugs frequently lead to this uncontrollable pattern of use. *Nicotine, cocaine and amphetamine, and heroin and other opiate drugs are highly addictive*, as many people who start using these drugs have great difficulty in stopping or regulating their use. Alcohol may be one step down in "addictiveness." While many people do develop addictive patterns of alcohol use, many more people drink alcohol without developing compulsive patterns of use. However, it is good to remember that there are more alcoholics in this country than cocaine, amphetamine, and heroin addicts combined. The reason is simple: Alcohol is freely available and socially acceptable, while these other drugs are illegal, socially unacceptable, and difficult to obtain.

What is the number one addiction concern for children? *Cigarettes.* Few people can "take or leave" cigarettes. This may be the addictive drug that people have the most trouble stopping. Cigarettes are freely available to the adult population, and children can easily get their hands on cigarettes.

A couple of drugs that you might have expected on the list above were not there. Marijuana was not, nor was caffeine or Valium and other sedatives. The reason is that while some individuals develop compulsive patterns of using these substances, most do not. Plenty of people use marijuana too much, and many people are concerned about their caffeine intake. However, the "craving" for coffee just isn't as strong as the craving for cocaine. People want to avoid withdrawal from caffeine, and they count on their daily wake-up cup of tea or coffee, but the chemical lure to use it is not as powerful.

Why do these drugs feel good? Although peer influences, family history, and many other social factors influence drug use, *every single person has the biological makeup to become a drug addict.* Why? Because every one of us has a neural pathway in our brain that is designed to help us feel pleasure. This "reward" pathway serves a very important purpose: It causes us to enjoy the activities that are life sustaining. This pathway is the reason that we enjoy sex, food with life-sustaining calories (the Big Mac attack lives here), and the process of seeking out and consuming these life-sustaining things. (We discuss this subject in more detail in Chapter 13, Stimulants.)

Research shows that all of the addictive drugs are able, one way or another, to activate this pathway. Drugs like marijuana and caffeine activate the pathway just a little if at all, while stimulants, opiates, and nicotine are especially good at activating it. So taking cocaine becomes a substitute for all the normal, life-sustaining things a person usually does. It replaces sex, eating, and interacting normally with the environment. Now it becomes easier to understand the allure. Heroin users often compare the "rush" they experience after injecting heroin to having an orgasm. This is no accident. While they don't actually have an orgasm, they experience a similar sensation of pleasure originating in the same chemical responses in the brain.

Obviously, the reward system is not the whole picture. Once people get into a pattern of using drugs, they often say that they really don't enjoy the drugs anymore, they are just trying to prevent the bad feelings of withdrawal. This is true, to an extent. For specific drugs, and heroin provides a good example, withdrawal happens between each dose and is physically uncomfortable. For other drugs, such as cocaine, withdrawal is not dramatic. However, after regular use of any addictive drug, another powerful process may occur. It is possible that the reward system may adjust, or become tolerant, so that normal pleasure is experienced only in the presence of the drug. You can view the process as the same as that occurring for nose drops, but it is happening in the pleasure centers of the brain.

6. How Does Drug Use Lead to Addiction?

Most people start using addictive drugs when they are teenagers. A desire for new experiences, a group of peers who provide a supportive environment, and the availability of drugs and opportunity to use them contribute to drug taking in teenagers. Inhalants are often the first psychoactive drug that kids take and are a perfect example of what typically happens with psychoactive drugs: *People use drugs because they work, and because they are available.* Inhalants can make you feel a little woozy, and they are immediately available to almost all children.

Cigarettes are an even more common starting point for psychoactive drug use. Almost everyone who smokes started smoking during their teenage years. Tobacco company advertising targeted at the teenage audience was no mistake. This is the age group that constitutes "entry-level" users. Studies of tobacco advertising have suggested that the intentional marketing of a "starter" brand of snuff, for example, represents a blatant attempt to lure children with a taste that in some way resembles candy.

One theory about drug taking is that there is a "gateway" through which teenagers pass that represents the start of an inevitable path to use of hard drugs. A lot of obvious factors contribute to drug use: (1) *lack of knowledge about the dangers,* (2) *availability and opportunity,* (3) *a peer group that is using the drug,* (4) *a natural desire to experiment,* and (5) *the desire to self-medicate bad feelings or avoid bad life circumstances.* Clearly, a complex set of factors leads to continued drug use—it is too simplistic to blame this process on the initial use of one drug.

Lack of knowledge about the dangers is where parents should start their education about drugs. That is why we wrote this book. We think that scare tactics are not necessary because the truth is scary enough! Therefore, the best protection any family has is knowledge and the clear communication of that knowledge. However, drug education alone does not stop drug taking. Over and over again, programs that focus just on drug facts fail.

Part of the reason that drug education alone fails to prevent drug use is the second factor we listed: availability and opportunity. It is one thing to listen to a police officer abstractly discuss the dangers of marijuana and quite another to see someone smoking a joint at a party and not be tempted to try it. While education can strengthen a teenager's resolve, limiting availability and opportunity certainly puts a practical damper on drug use. Proof of this fact is found in worldwide statistics on deaths due to alcohol-related diseases. In countries in which Islam is the dominant religion, deaths from cirrhosis of the liver are much lower than in other countries for the simple reason that this religion forbids use of alcohol. Of course, not everyone is perfectly observant, but a cultural approach that discourages drug use certainly helps. By "culture" we mean any group of people, ranging from a country to a school system to an individual family. Parents must examine their own attitudes on this point. The job of parents is to limit availability and opportunity, which is easily said and difficult to do. Furthermore, this challenges parents' own habits. The "do as I say and not as I do" command is a time-worn and often ineffective strategy. Availability and opportunity are areas where parents can have a big impact, but limiting children's access to drugs is a hard job.

Peer group influences are a tremendously important part of any child's environment. While we do not espouse the "parents are not important" point of view, we respect the power of peers. Adolescents look to their peer group for identity, and if drug using is part of that peer group, then it becomes important not just for social status, but for a child's own self-image. This is a factor that cannot be underestimated! Again, it is difficult to control your child's friendships, and attempting too much control may be unwise. But your knowledge of their friends gives you power. If you know your child's friends, you can make some informed judgments about how much freedom is appropriate with each particular friend. You cannot isolate your child, nor should you.

His or her independent decisions about friendships are part of becoming an adult. However, you don't need to disappear from the process either.

So far we have discussed lifestyle issues. However, basic biological factors probably do play a role in drug taking. Every human being has a natural desire for novel experiences. *Novel environments by themselves stimulate the reward system* in animals, and probably also do so in people. Everyone who gets pleasure out of travel can probably confirm this from their own experiences. Children especially have a natural desire to experiment with their behavioral state. Very young children will spin themselves around until they are dizzy. Our culture is one that emphasizes novel and arousing experiences, from scary movies to carnival rides to changing clothing styles. Some people have a particularly strong love of risk taking or thrill seeking. Sometimes this characteristic emerges early in childhood as daring childhood pranks—stealing from stores, pranks played on neighbors. Research indicates that risk takers have a higher than average tendency to take drugs. This should hardly be surprising. In middle school, cigarette smoking is a natural succession to the pranks of earlier childhood. Here is where understanding your own child will really help. If you have a child who avoids risk at any cost, he or she may well avoid drug-taking situations without your help. On the other hand, if you have a young daredevil, then you may need to be especially attentive.

People also take drugs to medicate bad feelings, and adolescence is a developmental stage that is full of negative feelings. Anxiety, depression, and untreated attention deficit disorder are all factors in drug taking in adults, and these are conditions that often go undiagnosed and untreated in children and adolescents. Therefore, professional help is vitally important for families in which children have already started taking drugs, or in families in which children are having emotional problems. Just "being tough" often will not solve the problem. You can restrict availability and opportunity, but you can't dictate feelings and should not underestimate their power in children and adolescents.

Finally, does that first taste of nicotine or marijuana cause permanent changes in the brain that lead to a "hunger" for drugs? This is one of the biggest fears that parents have. The answer is a qualified no. We do think that gradual adaptive changes in the reward system contribute to the process of addiction. However, this process probably takes some time, and a single experience is not enough to produce permanent changes in these neural circuits. Unfortunately, we don't have an answer about whether ten or one hundred experiences are necessary to produce such changes. However, people are quick learners—that's what our huge brain accomplishes. For a child or teenager who is anxious or depressed or unable to focus, if the drug makes him feel better, that alone will be a powerful incentive for drug use.

TALKING POINTS ABOUT DRUGS, DRUG TAKING, AND ADDICTION

• Any chemical or plant-based substance you put in your body intentionally to change your mental state or bodily function is a drug. This includes vitamins, antibiotics to cure infections, herbal teas, caffeine in sodas, and crack cocaine. The first step in educating your family about drugs is educating yourself and looking at your own drug-use habits. Consider the list of drugs just listed and whether it matches your own definition of drugs. This evaluation alone can be the source of a lively conversation with your kids. Count up the drugs you and your children take in a week (starting with that vitamin pill at breakfast). This provides the opportunity to explore the different reasons for taking drugs.

• Drugs enter the bloodstream, attach to a specific place in the body, and change how it works. This can mean fixing a system that isn't working, or taking a system that is working perfectly well and altering it. Most drugs affect the entire body, and many have unexpected side effects that can be harmful. You can use TV ads to initiate conversations with your children about how drugs travel throughout the body—many of these commercials correctly illustrated drugs being absorbed from the stomach and circulating throughout the body.

• Sometimes when we take a drug constantly, it stops working for us. This phenomenon is called *tolerance.* Or one's body may become dependent on what the drug does and work normally only if the drug is there. Then one is *dependent*, and taking the drug away causes *withdrawal.* You could discuss the caffeine headache we describe earlier in this chapter with older kids if you take caffeine yourself. However, you might do a simpler exercise. Since most of you wear a watch, think about how "naked" you would feel without your watch. You would be checking the spot on your wrist all day. Ask the kids about anything they do all the time that is so familiar that they would feel weird not doing it— like not wearing a favorite necklace that is worn every day. Or ask about something they have practiced a million times, like a particular sports move, so that not doing it seems stranger than doing it. You can explain that the inside of your body adapts the same way, and that is why drugs stop working sometimes and why you feel different if you stop taking them when you are used to them.

• The drugs that affect our behavior work just like other drugs, but they enter the brain and act on particular cells there. This is true of the many useful drugs that treat diseases of the brain, such as depression, anxiety, schizophrenia, and epilepsy, as well as of most "recreational" drugs. In talking with your children, you may need to explain to them the idea that drugs enter the brain just like they enter other parts of the body. We recently asked a group of high school students to list drugs that act on the brain. They gave a long list of abused drugs, but didn't think about caffeine or even prescription drugs used to treat disease. Explain to your children that they should think about their brain as an organ that they should keep healthy like their muscles or any other body part.

• Some people who take drugs feel compelled to repeat the experience over and over again. *Addiction* is this pattern of compulsive drug taking, without control, and despite bad consequences. Drugs that are addictive act on a part of the brain that causes us to feel pleasure. The drugs stimulate a system that usually is stimulated by life-sustaining activities, such as seeking out and consuming food, or finding a sexual partner. It is easy to explain even to a younger child how disruptive addiction can be by pointing out that when you are using these drugs, those desires "take over" that part of the brain, and you think only about the drug, not even about eating to keep yourself alive.

• How does drug use lead to addiction? Most people start using addictive drugs when they are teenagers. A desire for new experiences, a group of peers that provides a supportive environment, and the availability of drugs all play a role in initiating drug taking. There is no one reason for the progression of occasional drug taking into addiction. You can teach your kids lots of ways to avoid this progression—staying away from a "bad crowd," not starting to smoke (we think that cigarettes are the real gateway drug), and most important, being involved in activities that they enjoy. Studies show over and over again that kids who participate in activities that are important to them are much less likely to become involved with drugs. As kids enter adolescence, sometimes the old standards—baseball, scouting, piano lessons—seem like "little kids" stuff. You might be able to help them focus on more mature activities. Maybe they want to be in a rock band, be in a local theater group for kids, or join a church youth group. The important thing is that the activity must be something they enjoy and care about.

3. LEGAL ISSUES

The United States, along with much of the world, is engaged in a "war on drugs," and the legal system is the main weapon in that war. Although governments spend some money on education and drug treatment, by far the greatest expenditures are for legal interdiction, confiscation, and incarceration.

This enormous legal effort to control illicit drugs has resulted in a patchwork of state and federal laws that defies understanding. In some places, arrest for a marijuana cigarette may result in a simple citation like a traffic ticket; in other locales, a person could receive a felony sentence. If the differences in laws are not enough, you must also consider the discretion of the local prosecutor. Some enforce the letter of the law, while others simply won't prosecute minor drug-related offenses. You just never know, and neither will the child you are educating.

For most drugs other than marijuana, the issue is much simpler—possession and distribution results in a felony conviction. And all you have to do to be charged with the higher crime of "distribution" is give a drug to someone else. If you give a controlled substance to someone and he or she dies, you can be prosecuted under a little-known federal law that carries a mandatory minimum sentence of twenty years. So if a teenager gives an

Ecstasy pill to a friend and she has a bad reaction and dies, the federal authorities have the power to prosecute that teenager, even if it ruins her life. Kids need to know just how harsh the rules can be.

THE MOST IMPORTANT THINGS TO KNOW ABOUT LEGAL ISSUES

1. The laws governing marijuana possession and distribution are complex and vary from state to state.

With all the talk about legalizing marijuana, kids can easily get the impression that being involved with marijuana is not legally risky. Nothing could be farther from the truth. A simple marijuana charge can produce significant grief and expense for both parents and kids.

Some kids think that marijuana is no longer a legal issue because it is widely used and is being legalized for medical use in some places. First, although marijuana may be legal for medicinal purposes in a few places, its recreational use is illegal and may carry harsh penalties. Second, the federal government does not recognize the legality of marijuana for any purpose, so there is always the possibility that a person will be charged under federal law.

For many kids, getting marijuana is easier than getting alcohol—drug dealers don't card them. But kids should not conclude that it is legally safe just because the drug is so widely available. Many police officers charge a person with marijuana possession or distribution and then let the prosecutors make the final decision as to whether to prosecute. Meanwhile, there is an arrest, and a record of the arrest, so a defense lawyer needs to be hired. One never knows what the prosecutor will do. Even if the person is never convicted, the arrest record remains on the books and his or her family is stuck with the legal and emotional expenses associated with the charge.

2. There is a very fine line between drug possession and drug distribution (dealing), and it's easy to be charged with a felony.

The way the laws are written, a person does not have to be a major drug dealer to be charged with "possession with intention to distribute." Often the law simply specifies that if you possess a certain amount of a drug, then you are intending to distribute it, no matter what your real intentions were. These are almost always felony convictions, especially for anything other than marijuana.

When we were writing our first book, *Buzzed: The Straight Facts about the Most Used and Abused Drugs from Alcohol to Ecstasy* (W. W. Norton, 1998), we had a federal prosecutor explain distribution to our college-age research interns. He picked up a small pack of cocaine and gave it to one of the students, and then had her hand it to the other intern. Then he pointed out that she had just distributed cocaine and was subject to being charged with a very serious felony. Obviously he was just making a legal point, but the point is clear—you don't have to exchange money, just drugs; and simply holding a modest amount of a drug can, in the eyes of the law, indicate distribution.

3. For drugs other than marijuana, the laws are much more severe.

Children often don't realize that all drugs are not treated in the same way. For Ecstasy, GHB, cocaine, heroin, and many other drugs, possession can easily be charged as a felony.

4. Alcohol and nicotine are also drugs, and possession and distribution by minors is illegal.

Because of the way alcohol and tobacco products are treated by the media, kids often don't realize that it is illegal for them to possess these substances. However, because of the increasing sensitivity to drunk driving issues and nicotine addiction, the legal system is more attuned to enforcing these laws than most children realize.

TALKING WITH KIDS ABOUT LEGAL ISSUES

• Keep everything simple.

• Be sure to tell the truth when you talk with kids about the legal aspects of drugs.

• Because it is so common, marijuana is the best subject on which to tackle the legal issue. First, you should acknowledge that the drug is prevalent and that many kids buy it with relative impunity. Second, explain that despite its availability and possible use as medicine, it is illegal everywhere for recreational use.

• Next, explain how the legal system works—arrest, arrest record, hiring a lawyer, prosecution, and conviction. Children tend to see these kinds of issues as black and white, with no middle ground, so it is your job to explain the consequences of arrest, independent of conviction.

• You might call your local police department to get some information about how a marijuana charge is handled in your community. Do they issue a citation, or do they make arrests and bring offenders to the courthouse? Explain this procedure and be sure to emphasize that a lot of distress is associated with an arrest even if a person is not convicted.

• Familiarize yourself with the marijuana laws in your state. Point out that if a person is going to commit a crime such as marijuana possession, then he ought to know the consequences of that crime. Would he be expelled from school? Lose his driver's license? Be required to do community service? What about jail time? How much does a lawyer cost?

• Explain that just giving a drug to someone is "dealing" and that just holding a larger amount of the drug can cause a person to be considered a dealer in the eyes of the law. This fact allows you to make the point that the law can be much more serious than kids might think.

• Explain that becoming involved with "harder" drugs can be legally devastating. Children should understand that becoming involved with these drugs places them in the presence of people who are viewed by society as serious criminals. It's easy to get caught in a legal snare just by being in their presence. Even if they are innocent, extracting them from the legal process can be difficult and expensive.

• Explain to kids that talking and planning with others about getting drugs can be just as illegal as going to get them. (This relates to "conspiracy" laws.) An aggressive prosecutor can use these laws to obtain convictions for everyone involved in a group of drug users, not just those caught in possession.

• Kids need to know that possession of alcohol under age 21 is illegal almost everywhere in the United States and that possession of tobacco products under age 18 is illegal in most places.

• As with other drugs, distributing alcohol and tobacco to others is a higher-level offense. Many places, especially around colleges, are tightening the enforcement of the alcohol laws, and some high school kids are also being charged.

• In some places a conviction for underage possession of alcohol can result in loss of driving privileges. Check the laws in your area.

• For children of driving age, stress the very serious conse- quences of driving under the influence. These laws are extremely strict for people under 21. Many places have a zero tolerance pol- icy, meaning a person can have no alcohol in his or her blood if under the legal drinking age. Again, check your local laws and be sure your kids understand them.

4. ALCOHOL

Most people consider alcohol a normal part of the culture in Western societies. We use alcohol to celebrate, worship, relax, and commiserate. We turn to it to relieve anxiety, to "take the edge off," to suppress our inhibitions, and sometimes to sedate ourselves to the point that we no longer experience pain. The media flood us with positive messages about alcohol. So it comes as a shock to many people to talk about alcohol as a powerful drug. But that is exactly what it is.

Alcohol is the most widely used recreational drug in the United States, and most people underestimate how powerful it is. Because it is a toxic compound for many organs of the body, if it were being brought to market today as a legitimate drug, it is unlikely that it would be approved by the U.S. Food and Drug Administration for use without a prescription. Compared to many drugs, such as Valium, the difference between a recreational dose leading to drunkenness and a toxic dose leading to loss of consciousness or death is small.

So, as a parent, remember that when you use alcohol, you are choosing to use a powerful drug and that you are modeling the behavior for your children. Every time a child hears about someone he respects using alcohol, whether it be a sports figure, an older role model, or a family member, that child is learning about using recreational drugs.

As you talk with your children about alcohol, remember that they have been watching their family and their heroes all of their lives. So think about how they have seen alcohol used and what messages they may have received. If you feel that you have not been a great model, think about changing your behavior to reflect the way you would want your children to behave. If you do decide to change, tell your children that you are doing it. It will make an impression on them.

There are important points convey to children about this drug. Alcohol is legal, intensively advertised, and widely available, so there are bound to be many occasions when the subject of alcohol will come up spontaneously with children. You should seize these opportunities for a conversation about what alcohol is and what it does.

THE MOST IMPORTANT THINGS TO KNOW ABOUT ALCOHOL

1. Alcohol is the drug of choice in our society.

Alcohol is available to almost anyone who can walk outside their home and is accessible to many children from their parents' liquor cabinet. Children have no difficulty getting alcohol, and they need to understand that you know they have access to it, that you know that they will have the opportunity to use it, and that you are concerned. Whether or not they ever use alcohol, they will be in contact with it and will have to make decisions about its use.

Many parents underestimate the number of teens who drink and the amount of alcohol they use. Despite the laws and the best efforts of some parents, the latest available numbers we've found from the University of Michigan's "Monitoring the Future" project paint a rather disturbing picture. The table below shows the percentage of children, by grade level, who report using alcohol.

	8th-Graders	10th-Graders	12th-Graders
Used during past year	43%	65%	73%
Used in past 30 days	22%	41%	50%
Been drunk in past year	19%	42%	52%
Been drunk in past 30 days	8%	24%	32%
5+ drinks in a row in past 2 weeks	15%	25%	31%

While all of these numbers are cause for concern, perhaps the most striking are those related to having drunk five or more drinks in a row in the past two weeks. Five or more drinks in a row is the number that many researchers use to define "binge drinking," and it represents an amount of alcohol that can cause dangerously high blood alcohol levels. The fact that fully a quarter of tenth-graders reported this level of drinking during the past two weeks is a cause for concern.

So why do so many young people drink alcohol? Clearly there is no single answer to this question, but one factor that certainly plays a part is the fact that alcohol is legal for adults and is embedded in the fabric of our society. As a society, alcohol is clearly our "drug of choice." A quick look at popular magazines or television programming will show a huge number of very slick and attractive advertisements for alcohol—and these ads can be quite appealing to children.

Recent studies of drug use show that high school students, and even middle school students, decide about whether or not to use a drug based on how risky they perceive it to be and how well accepted it is by society. Given the high profile that alcohol has in our society it should come as no surprise that many young people feel it is a safe drug and choose to use it.

2. Alcohol makes people feel good (for a while).

The first effect one feels after a drink is a "buzz" that is slightly stimulating, relieves some anxiety, and reduces inhibitions. Within a few minutes after drinking (depending on how much food is in the stomach and the concentration of alcohol in the beverage) most people feel relaxed and pleasant and may become more talkative and outgoing—in general, less inhibited. Although alcohol is considered to be a "sedative" drug—one that produces sleepiness—people usually feel stimulated while the level of alcohol in the brain is increasing.

Alcohol makes people feel stimulated and "up" as the blood level rises. It enhances the effects of a brain chemical called GABA, which inhibits the activity of most brain circuits. The first circuits affected are those that cause us to feel anxiety and inhibition. It also indirectly promotes the release of the same chemical in the brain (dopamine) that is released by cocaine and other drugs that stimulate the brain. Dopamine produces a feeling of well-being, power, and confidence. There's more about this effect in the chapter on Stimulants.

However, the activation is soon replaced by sedation as the rising alcohol levels inhibit more and more circuits. As the amount of alcohol reaches its peak and begins to fall, most people feel mellow and sleepy and become withdrawn rather than sociable. Now the inhibitory effects of alcohol outweigh the stimulatory effects. During this time the drinker may become drowsy and depressed and may be motivated to drink more in order to "chase the high" felt just a little while before. Some young people who have consumed dangerously high amounts of alcohol report that they did so in order to continue to feel the way they did after their first drink or two.

3. Alcohol can be lethal if one drinks about four times the amount required for legal intoxication.

Many people do not realize that it is possible to die of a single alcohol overdose. Commonly, people associate the term "overdose" only with drugs like heroin or barbiturates, but alcohol can also kill if enough is consumed at one time. Because young people often are prone to binge drinking and many do not have much drinking experience, they are at particular risk for inadvertently stepping over the line to dangerous doses of alcohol. People die from alcohol poisoning because, at high concentrations, alcohol shuts down the parts of the brain that are critical for breathing and other automatic actions.

Even if the amount of alcohol does not reach a lethal level, there is still great danger. The body treats the alcohol as a poison and wants to get rid of it. Often at high alcohol levels a person may vomit. Unfortunately, high levels of alcohol paralyze a muscle that closes the trachea (windpipe) when we eat or drink—closing the trachea keeps water and food from going into our lungs. When an intoxicated person vomits, there is a real risk of asphyxiation from inhaling into the lungs the material that was vomited. Even if the person does not die immediately, there is a chance that material entering the lungs will cause a very serious, and sometimes fatal, lung inflammation or infection. (A student at our institution died like this very recently.)

How much alcohol does it take to put someone in danger of fatal alcohol poisoning? The fatal amount varies quite a bit from person to person, depending on body size and how quickly the alcohol is consumed. In general, any blood alcohol level above about 350 milligrams of alcohol per 100 milliliters of blood could represent significant danger. This level would be represented as "350 mg/dl" in a scientific report, and it corresponds to a reading of 0.35 on most breathalyzer machines.

A 150-pound male would achieve this level after quickly consuming 6.8 ounces of pure alcohol in an hour. He would get that much alcohol from about seven 2-ounce shots of strong bourbon. A 100-pound female would achieve this level after quickly drinking about four 2-ounce shots in an hour. Of course, it's possible to achieve a dangerously high blood alcohol level drinking beer or wine as well. For example, our 150-pound male would get to the dangerous range after drinking about twelve beers in an hour, and our 100-pound female would be in dangerous territory after about six and a half beers, or a little more than a six-pack.

When kids get themselves to dangerous blood alcohol levels, it is often because they are meeting a drinking challenge or playing a drinking game. These situations can be particularly dangerous because of strong pressure to "perform" in front of peers and because the game is usually a race to see who can be the first to guzzle a six-pack or a pitcher of beer.

Some people do not realize that alcohol can be mixed in ways that conceal its flavor or concentration, so a person can consume a lot very quickly without realizing how much alcohol is being taken in. In "Jell-O shots," for example, an alcoholic beverage such as vodka is mixed with Jell-O and frozen in ice-cube trays. Each cube, or "shot," can then be swallowed quickly without the burning taste of alcohol. Because of the ease with which they can be consumed, and the high alcohol concentration, Jell-O shots can quickly result in dangerous blood alcohol levels.

Most people don't know that if someone has been drinking more than about one drink in an hour, the level of alcohol in his or her blood continues to rise for a period of time even after the last drink. It takes a while for alcohol to enter the bloodstream, and the body can only eliminate it at a certain rate (about a drink an hour in the normal adult, less in smaller children). Once there is enough alcohol in the blood, any additional alcohol simply builds up and waits its turn for elimination. Meanwhile, it continues to bathe the brain and other body tissues.

The body's delayed absorption and slow removal of alcohol can mean serious problems for the recreational drinker. The first involves the classic "one for the road." Say a person has consumed enough alcohol that the body is eliminating it as quickly as possible. Then, believing (usually wrongly!) that she is able to drive home, she decides to have another drink before getting in the car. During the thirty-minute ride home, the alcohol from the last drink is absorbed and can elevate her blood alcohol level from one at which she might have been able to drive safely to one at which she clearly cannot. Many experts agree that it only takes a blood alcohol level of about 0.05 (50 mg/dl) to seriously impair the ability to drive a car.

The last "nightcap" can also prove dangerous if the person falls asleep while blood alcohol levels rise. A person who has a night of heavy drinking and then takes a few quick last drinks before falling asleep might not wake up.

4. Low doses of alcohol can impair a person's abilities.

A person can be significantly impaired by alcohol and not feel or appear so—even to a trained eye. In one study, only about 10 percent of people with a blood alcohol level around 50 mg/dl (sufficient in the opinion of many experts to significantly impair driving) appeared to be intoxicated when rated by trained observers. More strikingly, only about 65 percent of those people who had blood levels well in excess of the established legal limits for drunk driving appeared impaired to the trained observers in the study. Appearances can be very deceiving when it comes to alcohol.

As we mentioned above, the amount of alcohol that is necessary to impair the ability to drive a car is well below the limits that have been set to define a person as legally drunk. This is because driving a car requires a rather complex set of activities involving attention, concentration, coordination of movements, reaction time, judgment, and memory. The brain has to work a lot harder to do all of these things at once than it does when a person is quietly watching a movie or having a conversation with friends. And this is exactly the point—with a low dose of alcohol on board, impairments do not become obvious until sufficient demands are placed on the brain. So someone who has consumed only a modest amount of alcohol can actually be dangerously impaired in many situations.

5. The adolescent brain is different from the adult brain.

Nearly everyone seems to appreciate that adolescence is a unique time of life, but recent research suggests that alcohol affects adolescents differently than adults in some very important ways.

In the past, most parents could only tell teens that they shouldn't drink because it was illegal and/or because the parents told them not to. Neither approach ever carried much weight, judging by the staggering number of teens in the United States who drink. Now, however, some scientific findings can help change the discussion from an emotional one to one based on facts.

Not so long ago most people thought that development of the brain was virtually finished during early childhood and that little subsequent change took place until the effects of aging were

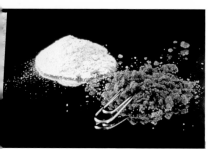
Mexican brown heroin and Southeast Asian heroin.

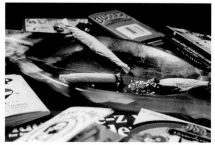
Marijuana rolled into cigarettes for smoking.

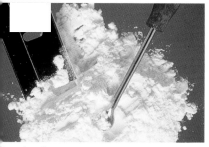
Powdered cocaine.

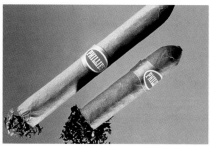
Hollowed-out cigars packed with marijuana, called blunts.

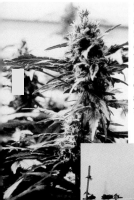
Marijuana abusers prefer the *colas,* or buds of the plant, because of their higher THC content. Leaves are discarded or used as filler.

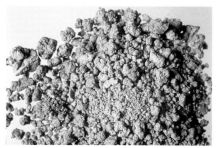
Mexican heroin.

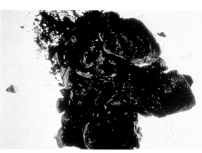
Marijuana buds hung out to dry.

Mexican black tar heroin.

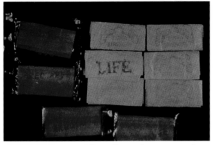
Heroin repackaged for sale on the streets of the United States.

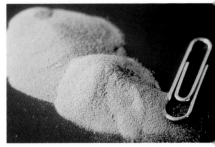
Morphine base.

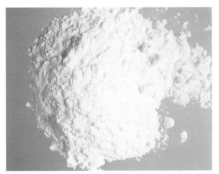
Highly refined Southeast Asian heroin.

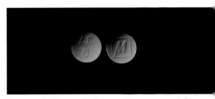
Demerol. Controlled ingredient: meperidine hydrochloride 100 mg.

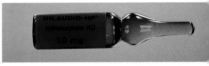
Dilaudid-HP injection. Controlled ingredient: hydromorphone hydrochloride 10 mg/ml.

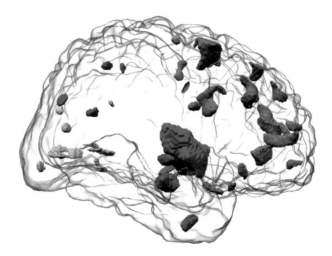
The adolescent brain is not mature. This is shown in the high resolution image created by subtracting averaged adult MRIs (magnetic resonance images) from averaged adolescent MRIs to show the areas of the adolescent brain that have not reached maturity. Green is the subcortical region, purple is the frontal region, red is the parietal region, yellow is the occipital region, and blue is the temporal region.

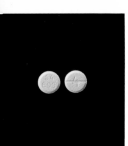

Hydromorphone hydrochloride. Controlled ingredient: hydromorphone hydrochloride 4 mg.

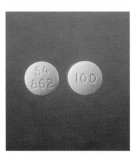

Oramorph SR. Controlled ingredient: morphine sulfate 100 mg.

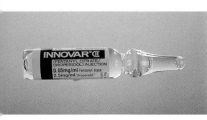

Innovar. Controlled ingredient: fentanyl citrate 0.05 mg/ml. Other ingredient: droperidol 2.5 mg/ml.

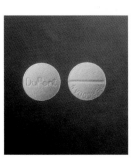

Percodan. Controlled ingredients: oxycodone hydrochloride 4.5 mg; oxycodone terephthalate 0.38 mg. Other ingredient: aspirin 325 mg.

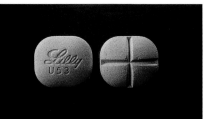

Methadone HCl diskets. Controlled ingredient: methadone hydrochloride 40 mg.

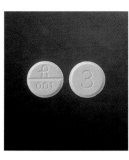

Acetaminophen with Codeine No. 3. Controlled ingredient: codeine phosphate 30 mg. Other ingredient: acetaminophen 300 mg.

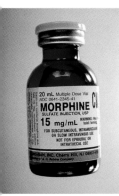

Morphine sulfate. Controlled ingredient: morphine sulfate 15 mg/ml.

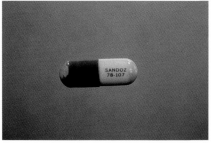

Fiorinal with Codeine. Controlled ingredients: codeine phosphate 30 mg; butalbital 50 mg. Other ingredients: aspirin 325 mg; caffeine 40 mg.

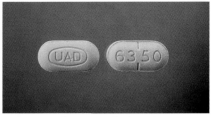

Lorcet. Ingredient name: hydrocodone bitartrate 10 mg. Other ingredient: acetaminophen 650 mg.

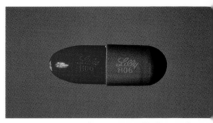

Darvon Compound-65. Controlled ingredient: propoxyphene hydrochloride 65 mg. Other ingredients: aspirin 389 mg; caffeine 32.4 mg.

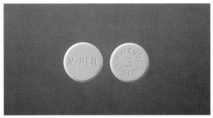

Tylenol with Codeine No. 3. Controlled ingredient: codeine phosphate 30 mg. Other ingredient: acetaminophen 300 mg.

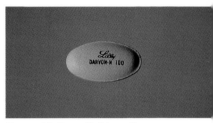

Darvon-N. Controlled ingredient: propoxyphene napsylate 100 mg.

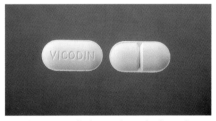

Vicodin. Controlled ingredient: hydrocodone bitartrate 5 mg. Other ingredient: acetaminophen 500 mg.

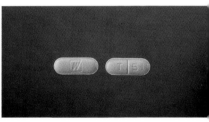

Talwin Nx. Controlled ingredient: pentazocine hydrochloride 50 mg. Other ingredient: naloxone hydrochloride 0.5 mg.

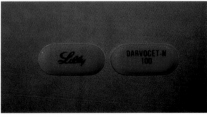

Darvocet-N 100. Controlled ingredient: propoxyphene napsylate 100 mg. Other ingredient: acetaminophen 650 mg.

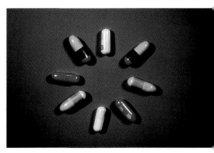

Depressants, or sedatives, widely prescribed to treat anxiety and insomnia.

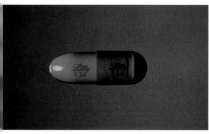

Amytal Sodium. Controlled ingredient: amobarbital sodium 200 mg.

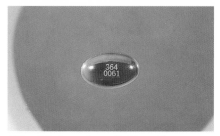

Chloral Hydrate. Controlled ingredient: chloral hydrate 500 mg.

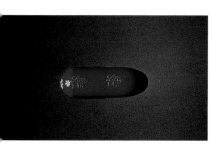

Nembutal Sodium. Controlled ingredient: pentobarbital sodium 100 mg.

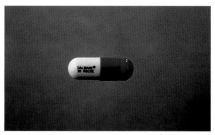

Dalmane. Controlled ingredient: flurazepam hydrochloride 30 mg.

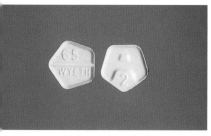

Seconal Sodium. Controlled ingredient: secobarbital sodium 100 mg.

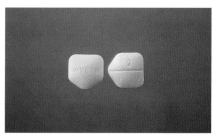

Equanil. Controlled ingredient: meprobamate 200 mg.

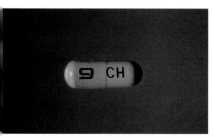

Ativan. Controlled ingredient: lorazepam 2 mg.

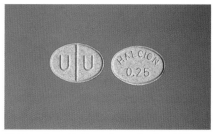

Halcion. Controlled ingredient: triazolam 0.25 mg.

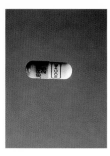

Librium. Controlled ingredient: chlordiazepoxide hydrochloride 25 mg.

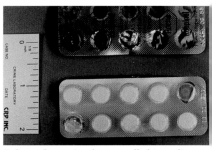

Rohypnol contains the controlled ingredient flunitrazepam hydrochloride. Pictured here is a 2-mg tablet with packaging. "Roofies," as they are known on the street, are sold inexpensively in Mexico. They are smuggled into the United States, where they have recently become a problem among American teens. The problem is rapidly spreading from the American Southwest to other parts of the United States.

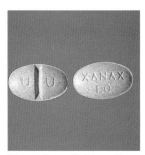

Tranxene. Controlled ingredient: clorazepate dipotassium 3.75 mg.

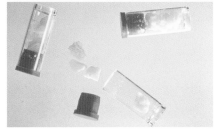

Crack, the smokable form of cocaine, provides an immediate rush.

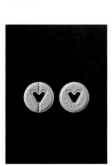

Valium. Controlled ingredient: diazepam 2 mg.

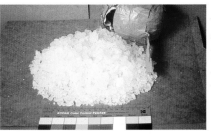

Ice, so named because of its appearance, is a smokable form of methamphetamine.

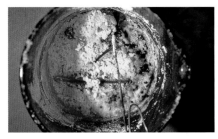

Crude methcathinone, or cat.

Xanax. Controlled ingredient: alprazolam 1 mg.

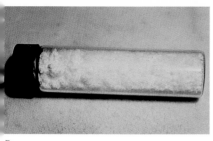

Pure cat.

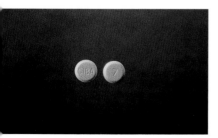

Ritalin. Controlled ingredient: methylphenidate hydrochloride 20 mg.

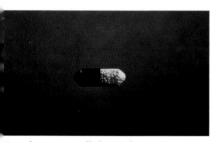

Dexedrine. Controlled ingredient: dextroamphetamine sulfate 5 mg.

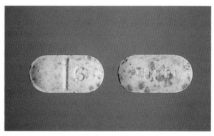

Adipex-P. Controlled ingredient: phentermine hydrochloride 37.5 mg.

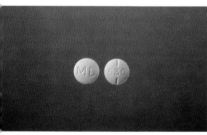

Methylphenidate hydrochloride. Controlled ingredient: methylphenidate hydrochloride 10 mg.

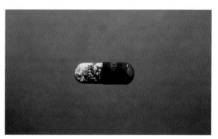

Fastin. Controlled ingredient: phentermine hydrochloride 30 mg.

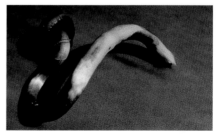

Ritalin. Controlled ingredient: methylphenidate hydrochloride 5 mg.

Psilocybin mushroom.

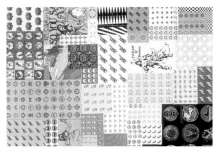

Collage of LSD blotter paper.

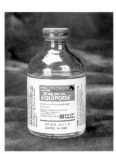

Counterfeiters duplicate packaging for black-market sales.

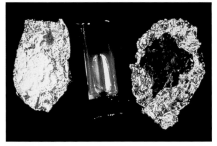

PCP is most commonly sold as a powder (left) or liquid (center), and applied to a leafy material such as oregano (right), which is then smoked.

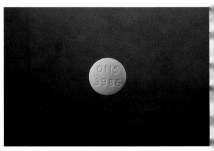

Android-25. Controlled ingredient: methyltestosterone 25 mg.

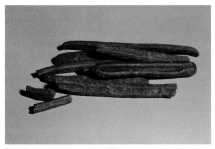

Black, resinous sticks of hashish.

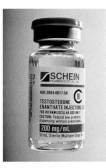

Testosterone. Controlled ingredient: testosterone 200 mg/ml.

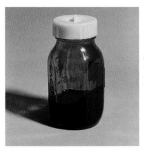

Amber, viscous hash oil.

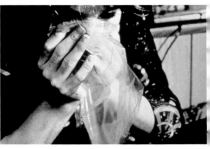

Sniffing an inhalant-soaked rag from a bag is a form of huffing.

observed. It has become clear that the brain continues to develop throughout childhood and adolescence, up to about the age of 20. One way in which the developing brain is different from the adult brain is in its ability to change in response to experience. An example of this type of change is learning. The young brain appears to be "built to learn." Since the young brain is in the process of making permanent connections between the nerve cells, the presence of any chemical during this period could change that "wiring" in unpredictable ways for the rest of a person's life.

Another fact is that the brain tends to change in response to the repeated use of a drug. As we explained in the chapter describing how drugs work (Chapter 2), the brain adapts to chemicals by modifying itself to reduce its sensitivity. This process is the basis for what we call drug tolerance. We have very little information about how well the brain "adapts" to repeated alcohol exposure during adolescence. Experience with other drugs suggests that it might even be *less* tolerant, which means the brain could be *more* affected over the long run.

The most recent research suggests that alcohol is a drug that affects the adolescent differently than it does fully mature people. In some ways alcohol is more powerful in adolescents, and in others it is less powerful. Studies using animal models found that alcohol impaired the activity of a brain chemical involved in learning much more potently in young animals than in mature animals. In fact, in the adolescent brain this activity was impaired by an amount of alcohol small enough to represent about one drink. This finding was reflected in experiments that tested the ability of young animals to learn under the influence of alcohol. Low doses that had no effect on adults seriously impaired the ability of the young animals to learn.

A recent study from our laboratories tested the influence of alcohol on learning in people between the ages of 21 and 29. The results were striking. Alcohol impaired learning much more in the people 21 to 24 years old than in those 25 or older. This result shows clearly that, even during young adulthood, alcohol has potent effects on learning. For legal and ethical reasons we could not do this type of research in teenagers, but our bet is that the effects would be even more noticeable in teens.

All of this seems to paint a rather simple picture—alcohol impairs mental function in young drinkers more than in adults, and thus teens shouldn't drink because their brains are more sensitive. But in at least one way the adolescent appears to be *less* sensitive to the effects of alcohol. Studies using animals have shown that high doses of alcohol are much less sedative in adolescents than in older animals. This suggests that alcohol may make young people less sleepy than adults.

Of course this doesn't make it any safer for teens to drink. It only means that adolescents may be able to drink more than adults before becoming sleepy enough to stop drinking. Moreover, the brain functions that control sleepiness aren't the same ones that control judgment and decision making. A teen may stay awake enough to function after drinking, but still make very bad decisions about what to do. A pharmacology professor of ours used to say, "A wide-awake drunk is still drunk."

What this research tells us is that adolescents have exactly the wrong pattern of sensitivities to alcohol. They may be able to drink more than adults without going to sleep, and they make get more of a buzz from alcohol, but they are also more vulnerable to the effects of alcohol on mental function.

6. Binge drinking is especially risky.

Children and adolescents (including college students) who drink often have five or more drinks in a row. This amount is defined in the scientific and medical literature as binge drinking for males. The number of drinks that constitutes a binge for females is four. According to the 1997 National Survey on Drug Abuse, more than 40 percent of the 11 million drinkers aged 12 to 20 in the United States engaged in binge drinking.

The reasons for binge drinking among young people are not entirely clear, but it's probably because they *really* like the buzz from the rising alcohol levels, and also because of the circumstances under which they consume alcohol. The fact that drinking is illegal for teens often obliges them to drink quickly in order to avoid getting caught, such as on the way to a party or during a brief time when their whereabouts are not known by parents. Whatever the reasons for it, binge drinking is a bad idea and should be a topic of conversation between parents and teens.

Of course, binge drinking involves consuming large doses of alcohol, and we have discussed the risks of lethal overdose above. But in addition to the physical dose of alcohol achieved during a binge episode, there are other social and emotional risks. For example, one study of college students who engaged in binge drinking showed that 63 percent had done something "under the influence" that they later regretted. Fifty-four percent of these students reported that they had the experience of forgetting where they were or what they did while drinking—a mentally compromised position that can lead to real danger. They also reported that their sexual behavior had been influenced by alcohol—41 percent said they had engaged in unplanned sexual activity while drinking, and 22 percent reported having engaged in unprotected sex.

In addition to the immediate risks associated with a given binge episode, evidence suggests that this *pattern* of drinking may be particularly bad for the brain. In one study, "social drinkers" were given tests of mental ability while they were *not* under the influence. It turned out that many of these people had mild to moderate deficits in mental functions. This is not surprising given what we know about the effects of alcohol on the brain over time. However, it was surprising that the single best predictor of mental impairment in the social drinkers was how much alcohol they drank per drinking occasion. People who drank more per occasion were more likely than others to show mental deficits, even if their overall lifetime consumption of alcohol was the same.

The brain is a sensitive organ. When a person drinks a lot in one sitting, abstains from alcohol for several days, and then binges again, brain activity gets bounced around like a yo-yo. It is powerfully suppressed by the alcohol, then "rebounds" into a hyperactive state as the first binge subsides. (This is the same phenomenon that causes adult or teen drinkers to wake up in the middle of the night feeling wasted.) When this pattern of suppression-rebound-suppression is repeated every few days, it may be particularly bad for the brain. Some evidence suggests that the "rebound" state may be directly damaging to nerve cells in the brain.

7. Other drugs can multiply the dangerous effects of alcohol, particularly those that cause sedation and sleepiness.

Some of the drugs that can compound the dangers of alcohol are:

- Valium (diazepam) and other sleep or anxiety medications
- Antihistamines or allergy drugs
- Cold medicines with the cough suppressant dextromethorphan
- Barbiturates (such as pentobarbital or phenobarbital)
- Recreational drugs (such as heroin or the date-rape drug GHB)

One of the most important facts about drugs is that their interaction can produce powerful, and often dangerous, effects.

Alcohol is a particular problem because it is so widely used that often people do not think of it as a potent drug and mistakenly take medicine or another recreational drug along with it.

Two opposing influences work on nerve cells in the brain—excitatory chemicals and inhibitory chemicals. The excitatory chemicals make the nervous system take action, and the inhibitory chemicals control the action so that the nervous system does not get out of control. It's like the accelerator and brake of an automobile. In general, alcohol suppresses the action of excitatory chemicals and enhances those that are inhibitory—it releases pressure on the accelerator and puts pressure on the brake. All of the drugs listed above put the brake on the brain. So, if one takes alcohol with a medicine or recreational drug that has one or both of these effects, then there is a real danger of a bad interaction. The interaction can take many forms, but one of the most dangerous is the suppression of life functions, such as breathing, at alcohol levels that would not normally cause a problem. Since many drinkers are not aware of this interaction, they think they can drink their usual amount, and then they find themselves in trouble.

People who drink must be especially cautious with medicines that are sold as "timed-release" capsules, often available over the counter for allergy relief or suppression of cold symptoms. A person might take a pill and then forget that this chemical is about to be released for the second or third time, have a drink, and suffer a bad reaction.

There are other reactions between alcohol and medicines. Even dose combinations that do not lead to breathing problems can result in profound impairment of movement, thinking, and judgment far beyond what would have resulted from the dose of alcohol alone. Often a pharmacist offers information about these hazards when a medicine is dispensed. For over-the-counter medicines, there is usually some warning on the package. However, the safest course is to remember that alcohol is a drug and that mixing drugs can produce serious problems.

TALKING WITH KIDS ABOUT ALCOHOL

• Find an example of an alcohol advertisement and talk about it with your kids. Point out that the company is trying to convince people to use alcohol and that they use powerful images to do so. The Budweiser frogs, for example, are funny, friendly creatures that capture attention and focus it on the beer. They also make it seem harmless—or as if it may make you goofy but not sick or in danger of getting hurt. Other ads use sex appeal, showing beautiful people having fun while drinking alcohol. Point out that the advertisements are not telling the whole story—if a person uses too much alcohol, she can put herself in danger or damage her body.

• Acknowledge that children who have never used alcohol may soon have the opportunity. The table earlier in the chapter shows that more than 40 percent of tenth-graders have drunk alcohol within the last month. This means that even if your child is not using alcohol, chances are she knows someone who is. So, what do you say? Acknowledge that peer pressure is important and that when her friends do something there is great temptation to follow along. But it is important for your child to make her own decisions. You can help her to do so by teaching her the facts about alcohol. The information in this chapter will help.

• Talk about the fact that people find alcohol attractive because it makes them feel good for a while, by activating parts of the brain that are there to make us feel good after doing things that are good for us, like eating. As we explain in the chapter on Stimulants (Chapter 13), the brain's reward system is present in humans and other animals to ensure that they behave in ways that will promote their survival. If you are comfortable talking about sex, explain that sex is a great stimulant of the reward system because it is necessary for survival of the species, and the brain is organized in a way to ensure that we want it. If it works better for you, talk about candy, other delicious foods, good smells, or winning at sports—anything that is pleasurable. Then talk about alcohol as an artificial chemical turn-on for this system—but a very powerful one.

• Make the point that repeated chemical activation of this system can cause people to crave that chemical and want to keep using it even if it hurts them.

• Explain that, in addition to activating the reward system, alcohol also turns off parts of the brain that are there to protect us—the anxiety centers that make us anxious and fearful in the presence of danger. They probably also keep us from doing things that we know are wrong. So when a person drinks, he may make decisions that he would not otherwise make.

• Think of some situations in which anxiety might be beneficial, and the potentially dangerous consequences of having that anxiety reduced by alcohol. Two excellent subjects are sex and reckless driving, but there are lots of other examples of risky behavior that people choose under the influence of alcohol.

• Explain that although some people use alcohol and other drugs to avoid the anxiety associated with painful parts of their lives, like a boring job, a bad relationship, difficult peer interactions, or general social stresses, the drug never changes the underlying situation, only the brain's response to that situation. Use candy as an example. Can eating more and more chocolate change a bad grade on a test?

• Acknowledge that we all want to change the way we feel from time to time. All of us suffer disappointments and pain, or enjoy being giddy and happy, but using chemicals to achieve mood changes is only a very short-term solution.

• There is probably no more important conversation to have with children than one in which the dangers of alcohol poisoning and fatal overdose are clearly and openly discussed. Get started by explaining that our brains not only give us the ability to think and feel, but also control many of the important functions of our bodies that we do not think much about, such as breathing and temperature regulation. If the brain stops maintaining these functions, even for a brief time, a person will die. Talk about the brain as the central processor in a computer—take it out and, while some things might still operate, the computer is completely dysfunctional.

• Explain that when a person drinks a lot at one time he may put enough alcohol into his brain to shut down basic body functions. There are no clear warning signals to the drinker when the blood alcohol level is about to move into dangerous territory, and even if there were, he might be too impaired to notice or care about them. Once a person has drunk enough to pass out, he is helpless, and if the blood-alcohol level then rises to lethal levels he will die.

• Remind kids that vomiting when drunk is dangerous, because they may inhale what they vomit. It's an unpleasant thought, but it makes an impression. Kids think that vomiting will help get rid of the alcohol in their bodies, but it only clears the last little bit they have consumed—so choosing to vomit is a bad idea. The best idea is to never drink enough alcohol to come anywhere near a lethal level or one that causes vomiting.

• Go to your police department or local Mothers Against Drunk Driving (MADD) chapter and get a chart that tells you how many drinks it takes to get to various blood alcohol levels for people of different weights. You can also find blood alcohol level charts for men and women, published by the U.S. government, at the following internet address: http://www.health.org:80/nongovpubs/bac-chart/index.htm. Then use the charts to calculate exactly how many drinks it takes to get to a level of 0.35 and how many it takes to get legally intoxicated. This is absolutely crucial information for kids to have; we recommend that you be sure they understand how many beers, glasses of wine, and shots of hard liquor make up these levels.

• Caution your child to never drink on a dare or consume beverages that are made to mask the flavor of high alcohol concentrations. College fraternities and sororities are often famous for their "punch" recipes, which hide the taste of alcohol. These concoctions often contain very high concentrations of alcohol but can be consumed painlessly and result in high blood alcohol concentrations very quickly.

• Let your child know that if he's been drinking and begins to feel very sleepy, or to have trouble speaking, walking, or focusing his vision, he is at risk and should get help. It is critical to let your child know that *you* are available to help no matter what. The last thing you want is a child in trouble to fail to call for help because he is worried about the consequences of his behavior. To some, this may seem like giving permission to drink but that is not the case. It is possible to be very clear with a child that you do not want him to drink and still acknowledge that occasionally there will be times when expectations may not be met. Make it clear that under those circumstances the first priority is his safety—and he should feel perfectly comfortable with calling you or anyone else for help.

• We recommend that a family "contract" be established to make these issues clear. Mothers Against Drunk Driving (MADD) has produced a CD-ROM (available at http://keytalk.madd.org/thekey), which is designed to help families with teens establish a contract about driving and drinking expectations. Each family will have its own expectations and rules, but whatever yours are, it is very important that all the family members understand them clearly, so that the contract provides a safety net for kids if they happen to get into trouble.

• A physical example is a good way to make the point that a little alcohol can impair performance. Think about a person with a minor illness or injury—say a twisted ankle. This injury probably would not make a kid feel much different while sitting at the dinner table or even walking around the house. But ask her to run outside and play in the neighborhood soccer game, and the mild ankle sprain would have a big impact on performance. A little bit of alcohol can be like a minor injury, not likely to be a bother until you try to do something more complicated than sitting around, and then the effects can be dangerous.

• Continually remind the child how unique and special his brain is. Tell him that his brain is still growing and changing and that this in some ways gives him a great advantage. He can learn more quickly and retain more information. That's why our society educates people at his age. But the very differences that give him advantages also hold additional risks. A changing brain is a vulnerable brain, and any disruption of the process of change could have long-term implications for how the brain works in the future.

• Point out that alcohol affects the chemicals that promote learning. Remind him of the stories he has heard about people being so drunk that they forgot what happened to them. Explain that this occurred because the learning chemicals were blocked. Let him know that the most recent research suggests that adolescents may be much more vulnerable to those effects than are adults.

• Explain that although alcohol might make an adult feel sleepy after a couple of drinks, kids may not feel so sleepy after the same number of drinks. However, that doesn't mean that alcohol is not impairing their physical activity, judgment, or coordination. In fact, they may be more "buzzed" than grownups by this drug.

• To explain alcohol withdrawal, stand a small spring upright on a table and point out that it stands up because it is neither compressed too tightly nor stretched in a way that makes it fall over. Now slowly compress the spring using a finger or pencil. When the spring is released it does not just return to its starting position, it "springs" upward and flies off the surface because of the released pressure. Explain that when brain activity is suppressed by a lot of alcohol, and then this pressure is released as the alcohol gets eliminated from the body, the brain becomes hyperactive for a time, just as the spring did when released. The cells of the brain can be damaged by this type of hyperactivity, and binge drinking is exactly the kind of drinking pattern that can create it.

• Be a model for healthy behavior. If you consume alcohol regularly, make a point of telling your children that you avoid using it when you are taking other medicines, unless the pharmacist or physician has told you that it is permissible. Talk about it. Tell them that you are not having wine or some other beverage because you are concerned about an interaction. Look at a package label or insert that comes with a medicine and point out the warnings about interactions with alcohol. If you feel it would be effective, ask your pharmacist or physician to explain this concept to your children.

• Talk about the fact that alcohol is a drug. Explain to your kids the concept of alcohol as a chemical that slows down the activity of the nervous system—that's why people like it, it suppresses the anxiety centers. Explain that many other drugs also suppress the nervous system like alcohol does—for example, cold and allergy medicines with antihistamines, cough suppressants with dextromethorphan, and anxiety-suppressing drugs such as Xanax or Valium. Use this opportunity to point out that even allergy medicines are drugs that affect their brains. It is also an opportunity to bring up the point that things we think of as part of a meal (like coffee and wine) are also drugs.

• Explain that you know some people use alcohol and other recreational drugs together. You do not have to be a drug expert to have this discussion, because it is a safe bet that mixing alcohol with any sedating drug (anxiety suppressants, antihistamines, sedatives, or opiates) will strengthen its effects. Caution kids that many drug interactions with alcohol can be unexpected and life-threatening and should be avoided.

5. CAFFEINE

Without question, caffeine is the most available mind-altering substance in the lives of children. It is in soft drinks, teas, coffees, some over-the-counter medicines, and even candy. For many adults, caffeine has become a routine part of each day, and we accept this as normal. What we might not recognize is that many children consume significant doses of caffeine each day too, though neither they nor their parents realize it.

Caffeine in moderation is perfectly safe. However, at high levels it is a powerful stimulant of the central nervous system—so powerful, in fact, that an overdose can produce epileptic seizures. It's even used to promote seizures in electroconvulsive therapy for depression. So it's a drug to take seriously.

Caffeine, and similar compounds such as theophylline (an asthma medicine) and theobromine, work by suppressing the effect of a brain chemical called adenosine. Adenosine is one of the most important chemicals for calming the brain. When it is not working properly, the brain becomes extremely excitable and normal stimuli can evoke greater responses.

At normal dietary levels, caffeine can increase the heart rate and blood pressure, as well as provide the lift or buzz that people really like. It's great for staying awake when you need to or just for being a bit more alert in boring situations.

Research clearly shows that, for adults, normal caffeine consumption (a couple of soft drinks or cups of coffee per day) is reasonably safe. At about twice those levels, problems with blood pressure and anxiety begin for some people. Too much caffeine makes people jittery, anxious, and even nauseous—all symptoms of overstimulation of the central nervous system.

THE MOST IMPORTANT THINGS TO KNOW ABOUT CAFFEINE

1. Caffeine is the most readily available psychoactive drug in our society.

Anybody can get caffeine anywhere—there are no legal restrictions for anyone of any age. It is in foods and drinks that children regularly consume. Most childern's caffeine intake is through soft drinks and tea. A look at some soft drink advertising shows that the buzz associated with caffeine is part of the appeal. You can see images of kids drinking certain soft drinks, playing hard, and having fun. These are effective images and would not be used if they didn't influence behavior.

2. Caffeine levels vary considerably between different products.

Here are some estimated caffeine levels for various foods and medicines.

Coffees—Average Caffeine Concentration

Drink	Milligrams
Dripped robusta coffee (8 oz)	150
Dripped arabica coffee (8 oz)	100
Percolated robusta coffee (8 oz)	110
Percolated arabica coffee (8 oz)	75
Instant coffee (8 oz)	65
Decaffeinated coffee (8 oz)	3
Espresso (and espresso-based drinks) made from arabica beans (1.5–2.0 oz.)	90

Teas—Average Caffeine Content

Drink	Milligrams
Brewed tea, domestic brand	
5-minute brew time	40 (20–90)*
1-minute brew time	30
Brewed tea, imported brand	
5-minute brew time	60 (25–110)*
1-minute brew time	45
Iced tea (12-oz glass)	70

*Depending on the particular brand tested

Soft Drinks—Average Caffeine Concentration

Drink	Milligrams
Canada Dry Jamaica cola	30
Coca-Cola	46
Dr Pepper	46
Mello Yello	53
Mountain Dew	54
Pepsi-Cola	38

Over-the-Counter Drugs—Caffeine Concentration

Brand Name	Milligrams
COLD REMEDIES	
Coryban-D	30
Dristan	16
Triaminicin	30
DIURETICS	
Aqua-Ban	100
PAIN RELIEVERS	
Anacin	32
Excedrin	65
Goody's Powders	33
Midol	32
Vanquish	33
STIMULANTS	
Caffedrine	200
No Doz	100
Vivarin	200

3. Caffeine has powerful short- and long-term effects on the body.

By increasing the excitability of circuits in the brain, caffeine stimulates centers that control both physical and psychological states. It is astounding how many body systems are affected by caffeine. The heart is stimulated, the kidneys produce more urine than usual, breathing becomes more rapid and airways are opened, and even the blood vessels of the eye are constricted. Caffeine increases responsiveness to stressors because it increases the amount of adrenaline circulating in the blood.

Caffeine affects several brain processes. Like all stimulants, it helps people to pay attention and focus on a task. It stimulates the part of the brain that keeps us awake, and it produces a mild euphoria that people really enjoy. At higher doses, it activates brain areas that produce anxiety, fear, and panic. Often, people with anxiety problems and those who have lots of stress in their lives find that they feel much better after they reduce their caffeine intake.

Caffeine can also have long-lasting effects on the brain. With regular use (every day or so), the brain adapts to the presence of caffeine by changing its chemistry. It begins to depend on the presence of caffeine to maintain its normal state for many functions. If a person stops using caffeine, all of the processes that have adapted to caffeine suddenly are out of sorts. It can take many days for them to re-establish normal characteristics.

You may have experienced this effect if you are caffeine-dependent. Remember missing that cup of coffee on Saturday morning and then getting the "headache from hell"? Remember how listless and depressed you felt? Then, if you remembered to get some coffee, remember the tremendous buzz you got? Well, that's a drug at work. Your brain became tolerant to caffeine, it missed it when you forgot your coffee, and it rebounded when you finally got around to getting some caffeine.

Should Kids Be Allowed to Use Caffeine at All?

Caffeine is a powerful drug that affects many brain systems, so should a developing brain be exposed to it? Right now there are no scientific studies that specifically answer this question. However, we are beginning to see some studies indicate that the developing brain may be particularly susceptible to some drugs, particularly alcohol. Everything we know as neurobiologists tells us that chronic use of any drug during brain development has the potential to change that development. Clearly, lots of kids use caffeine and seem okay. *We recommend that parents pay attention to how much caffeine kids are getting to ensure that they are not having trouble sleeping or becoming anxious.*

TALKING WITH KIDS ABOUT CAFFEINE

• Tell kids that caffeine is a drug and that it is present in many beverages they consume.

• Make a list with your children of the beverages and medicines they and their friends consume that contain caffeine (you can refer to the tables above). Explain that, over the course of a day, they may get caffeine from multiple sources and that it all adds up.

• Estimate how much caffeine is consumed each day. Point out that doses as low as about 50 mg can have psychoactive effects on adults, and since children's bodies are smaller, less caffeine is required to produce these effects. Explain that a dose of caffeine that might make an adult feel pleasantly alert can make children feel jittery and anxious simply because it amounts to a higher level of caffeine.

• Point out that caffeine is added deliberately to some soft drinks in order to enhance their appeal. Some manufacturers say that this is done for flavor, but clearly the stimulant effects of the drug must be part of the appeal. Emphasize that some food manufacturers are choosing to include caffeine as an ingredient because they think it will make their product sell better.

• Reflect on your own use of this drug and how you talk about it. Do you often talk about your "dependence" on caffeine for waking up in the morning or staying alert at night? Do you talk about the pleasant caffeine buzz that you get after drinking coffee or soda? If so, you may be sending the message that it's okay to use a drug to change your behavior and feelings. These can be very powerful messages for children and have implications for how they think about other drugs as well.

• Younger children will have a hard time understanding that caffeine regulates so many body functions. Although they certainly experience these effects, they probably won't recognize them unless they are using a tremendous amount of the drug. The best thing an adult can do is simply tell them that all these body processes are altered by caffeine, especially those that change their psychological state. Tell them you know caffeine can make them feel differently (maybe up, maybe not) even though they may not be able to describe the difference. Tell them that the fact caffeine can create these changes means that it is a powerful drug and is affecting their brains.

• With older kids you can talk about all of the body functions caffeine regulates. Acknowledge that it makes people feel good, and explain how that happens. Be sure to talk about its potential for producing anxiety and making stressful times worse.

• Older kids can also understand that the brain adapts to the repeated use of a drug and that caffeine is no exception. Warn them that regular use can result in real dependence.

• Sleep is a big issue for all children. Don't forget that caffeine can suppress the onset of sleep or impair the quality of sleep for anyone, young or old. As we discuss in the chapter on marijuana (Chapter 8), the information the brain acquires during the day is permanently encoded during sleep at night. Disrupted sleep diminishes learning.

6. HALLUCINOGENS

No single drug, or group of drugs, makes up the category of hallucinogens. The one characteristic they all share is that they change thinking, mood, and perception. Although the likelihood of fatal overdose is remote for most hallucinogens, a few can be quite dangerous—even in low doses. But even those drugs that have little overdose risk can be harmful in the wrong hands or under the wrong circumstances.

Hallucinogens have been a part of human culture for millennia. Both ancient and modern peoples have used them in religious and healing rituals. In some cultures, the community healer or shaman may use them to enhance his ability to fulfill his role in the community. In other cultures, hallucinogens are used in a spiritual or intellectual rite of passage.

This theme is consistent with how the use of hallucinogens has been perceived by some in the twentieth century as well. In the 1950s, hallucinogens were famously studied by Harvard psychologists Timothy Leary and Richard Alpert (later known as Baba Ram Dass). They were intrigued with the apparent capacity of psilocybin and LSD to promote a state of contemplation and enhanced self-awareness. Hallucinogens were viewed as potential psychotherapeutic aids and as potential keys to unlock the secrets of how the mind works. On the other side of the social divide that was developing in the United States in those years, the CIA was also intrigued with hallucinogens and conducted its own experiments. The motivation for those experiments was perhaps less clinically or spiritually inspired, but they were based on the same awareness that hallucinogens are powerful drugs that can affect some of the most subtle ways in which people think, feel, and perceive the world.

It is important to note that the purely recreational use of hallucinogens that seems to characterize their current popularity is a relatively new phenomenon. Many of today's users think of these drugs simply as a way to enhance a party buzz, not as the serious business that they have historically represented. This casual attitude toward hallucinogens can result in underestimating the power of these chemicals.

THE MOST IMPORTANT THINGS TO KNOW ABOUT HALLUCINOGENS

1. There are many different hallucinogens.

Almost all of the hallucinogens alter the way a person perceives the world, thinks, and feels emotionally. But they do these things in different ways—some of which are more dangerous than others. The most familiar drugs are the *LSD-like hallucinogens*—LSD, psilocybin mushrooms, DMT (dimethyltryptamine), and mescaline (from the peyote cactus). All of these drugs are taken by mouth, so the onset of the effects is relatively slow. During the first thirty minutes a person may experience dizziness, nausea, and anxiety. Next, vision is affected, and feelings of "unreality" and incoordination are experienced. A person may feel detached from his surroundings and even separate from his own body. One to two hours after taking the drug, the peak effects are felt, which include substantial changes in visual perception with wavelike motions in the field of vision, euphoria, and a feeling of slow passage of time. It can take up to twenty-four hours for the brain to return to normal. Although these effects can lead to potentially dangerous lapses of judgment, there is little risk of death from overdose with these drugs.

This is not the case for the *belladonna alkaloids,* such as Jimsonweed, deadly nightshade, and mandrake root, which contain the chemicals atropine and scopolamine. These chemicals work on a chemical system that controls not only mental functions but also the heart, the lungs, and body temperature. The name belladonna (or "beautiful woman") came about because the drugs dilate the pupils, which people find attractive. These drugs produce a strong delirium (disorientation) that often includes the sensation of flying, but they also produce amnesia so that a person might have only a vague recollection of the experience. These drugs can be deadly because they interfere with vital body processes.

PCP (phencyclidine) and *ketamine* (Special K) represent a different category of hallucinogens: painkillers that work by detaching a person from his own feelings. Ketamine does not suppress the pain directly like morphine does; rather, it creates a psychological detachment from the pain, so that a person or animal ignores the pain. It is used in treatment for animals and occasionally children, but it is not used for adults except in rare circumstances, because the hallucinations it produces are unpleasant. PCP is even more complicated because, in addition to hallucinations, it is also a stimulant and a morphine-like painkiller. So a person using PCP is hallucinating, feeling no pain, and overstimulated, which makes this drug, like ketamine, especially dangerous. Unlike the LSD "group," it is possible to take enough PCP or ketamine to die. They are also dangerous when taken with alcohol.

2. Some hallucinogens can "unmask" underlying mental health problems.

One of the myths about hallucinogens is that they can make some people permanently "crazy." The truth is that casual use of hallucinogens does not *cause* mental illness per se, but some people with a family history or predisposition toward mental illness may be more likely to experience symptoms while using these drugs. This distinction is best illustrated by an experience that one of us, Scott Swartzwelder, had some years ago. Scott had become known among the students at his university as a professor who taught about the brain and drugs. One day he received a phone call from the Dean of Students. She was in the emergency room with a student who had been brought in by some friends and was behaving in a bizarre way. He was refusing any medical attention until he could speak with Scott—though Scott did not know him at all. On arriving at the ER, Scott found the young man in a treatment room refusing to allow the technician to attach small electrode leads to his chest to monitor his heart. He believed that the wires were attached on the other end to a CIA monitoring facility because his thoughts were the subject of great government interest. As soon as Scott introduced himself, the student said that he was quite relieved because he was certain Scott was the only person in the world who could possibly understand the depth of his thoughts. He told Scott that he had taken many hits of LSD during the past few days. His speech was pressured and rapid, his ideas were grandiose, and he jumped from one idea to another quickly and with little sensible connection. Scott agreed to talk with him if he would allow the medical personnel to treat him. The young man accepted treatment and was found to be physically stable. Scott asked him to continue to cooperate and to let Scott know how he was doing in a few weeks. He agreed.

About a week or so later Scott learned that the student was

doing fine, but that he had received a psychiatric work-up and was diagnosed with bipolar disorder (formerly called manic depression). People in the manic phase of this disorder can become psychotic (i.e., unable to tell the difference between what is real and what is purely a product of their own thinking), as the young man's symptoms had indicated. When the medical team dug a little deeper, it turned out that there was a history of bipolar disorder in his family, so he was put on medication to diminish the chances of the psychotic symptoms reemerging. He will likely need psychiatric consultation periodically for the rest of his life, though he might not always require medication.

Did the use of LSD give him bipolar disorder? Certainly not. But on the other hand we'll never know if the symptoms of the disease would ever have emerged had he not shaken up his thought processes with the drug. This story is not so uncommon. It illustrates how hallucinogens can promote the expression of psychotic symptoms in some people.

3. Hallucinogens can cause flashbacks.

"Flashbacks" are unanticipated reexperiences of some of the aspects of a hallucinogenic trip long after the drug is out of the body. They may include visual disturbances or other "memories" of the drug experience. Flashbacks are much more common among people who have used hallucinogens heavily. Flashbacks can persist for many years, perhaps for life. They do not take the form of a full-blown trip, but rather are simple visual disturbances such as trails of light or wavering borders of images. We believe that this problem might reflect permanent changes in the way the brain processes visual information. The medical name for this is "post-hallucinogen perceptual disorder," and there are even support groups for victims of it. The problem can range from the trivial to the debilitating and can cause anxiety or depression. Unfortunately, there is no way to know who will experience the problem. We also don't know whether children are particularly susceptible, but given that their brains are still developing, there may well be an added risk.

TALKING WITH KIDS ABOUT HALLUCINOGENS

• Emphasize that many different kinds of drugs cause hallucinations. Somebody might simply ask a child if he wants to "trip" without naming the drug, so he must understand that the effects he could experience might be vastly different depending on which drug is offered.

• A trip can last a long time—in the case of LSD, up to a day—and during that time a person's ability to make good decisions can be very impaired. It is important that a person not be left alone in this state.

• All hallucinogenic drugs seriously impair judgment. This fact is the basis of the stories about people on LSD thinking they can fly if they jump off a balcony. Teach children that their minds control what they do and that when they are impaired by drugs they may do very dangerous things they would never do otherwise.

• A child should understand that the most physically dangerous hallucinogens are PCP, ketamine, and the belladonna alkaloids, which can alter life-sustaining body functions.

• Using hallucinogens, even one time, can cause terrifying experiences. A child may have heard of "bad trips," but for some people the experience can have long-lasting and frightening effects. Explain that everyone's brain is unique and that some appear to be wired in ways that make them more vulnerable than others to the effects of hallucinogens. For these people, hallucinogens can be very dangerous—leading to a long-lasting state of confusion that might require powerful medicines to control.

• Emphasize that it's impossible to predict who might be vulnerable to a severe reaction. If you know that the child you're talking with has a personal or family history of mental illness (particularly any mental illness that can involve psychosis, such as schizophrenia, bipolar disorder, or depression with psychotic features), she may be at substantial risk of triggering such an illness with hallucinogen use even if she's fine right now.

• Your approach should be entirely nonjudgmental in regard to mental illness. A personal or family history of mental illness is a delicate point. It is important to not throw this in a child's face in a way that makes her feel inferior or stigmatized. Explain that a person's history does not determine who she is or what she can become, but that it does provide an opportunity to make more informed choices, including those related to drug use.

• Teach the child that using hallucinogens can put him at risk for later, unwanted replays of some of the hallucinogenic experiences. Explain that these could come at any time and are outside of his control. You might want to do some research on the internet and read what people have written about this problem and, if appropriate, share that information with the child.

7. INHALANTS

nhalants are one of the first drugs that kids try, probably because they are so accessible. They're in the garage, under the kitchen counter, and available in every grocery store. They represent a very mixed group of chemicals ranging from cigarette lighter fluid to medical-grade nitrous oxide. In fact, the only thing all these chemicals have in common is that they are inhaled and they alter consciousness. This is a very easy group of drugs to understand because it breaks down into two categories: *industrial chemicals,* which were never intended for human use, and *nitrous oxide.*

We are continually amazed by the kids' strong desire to alter their consciousness. They go to such extremes as inhaling gasoline, paint thinner, lighter fluid, and a host of other industrial chemicals. One common factor to all of these industrial chemicals is that they are volatile and thus can easily be inhaled or "huffed" from a container or a soaked rag. Another common factor is that they are all extremely toxic to most organs in the body. Serious solvent intoxication resembles that of alcohol, with muscular incoordination, headache, abdominal pain, nausea, and vomiting. Some users describe changes in their perception of objects or time and/or have delusions or hallucinations involving any of the senses. Muscular incoordination occurs as toxicity levels increase, along with ringing in the ears (tinnitus), double vision, abdominal pain, and flushing of the skin. If a person inhales more, vomiting, loss of reflexes, cardiac and circulation problems, suppression of respiration and, possibly, death can be the result. Long-term use of inhalants can damage the heart, lungs, kidneys, liver, blood, and many other organs, in addition to the nervous system. *The bottom line is this: These chemicals were never intended for human use, they are extremely toxic, and you should do everything you can to keep kids away from them.*

Nitrous oxide is a medical anesthetic gas and it is a bit safer. We talk about that below.

THE MOST IMPORTANT THINGS TO KNOW ABOUT INHALANTS

1. All of the industrial chemicals kids use are extremely unsafe.

Kids use gasoline, lighter fluid, paint thinner, typewriter correction fluid, marking pens, acetone, toluene, spray paint, hair spray, and hundreds of others. Every one has its problems. If there were ever an area in which it is appropriate to make blanket statements, this is it. Never designed or tested for human consumption, these chemicals damage the brain, heart, liver, and kidneys, and they probably promote a wide variety of diseases. In addition, some of them do mechanical damage to body tissues, while others leave toxins around for years. They should be treated as poisons and kept in a locked area that is inaccessible to kids.

2. Kids die from inhalant use in different ways.

Studies show that inhalants kill by suppressing breathing, by producing toxic reactions in the body, and by causing kids to have fatal accidents. Some inhalant users have even committed suicide, although we're not sure of the role the drugs played in these deaths. A particularly tragic problem is *sudden sniffing death.* Some inhalants sensitize the heart to the effects of adrenaline, so any surprise that sends a surge of adrenaline to the heart might cause it to become arrhythmic and stop functioning. Typically this can happen when a kid is hidden away sniffing a chemical and he is discovered by an adult who startles him.

3. Nitrous oxide is much safer, but kids still get in trouble with it.

Nitrous oxide is a gas used in medical procedures to induce sedation, and it's also used in whipped cream containers to fluff up the cream. It's far less toxic than other inhalants, but kids can die from oxygen deprivation. Many people have had nitrous oxide in the hospital or dentist's office and know it produces a mild buzz, sedation, and pain relief. It's a lot like being quite drunk from alcohol. It's not particularly toxic, and although a few people become dependent on it, by and large it's very safe if properly used. The problem is that kids sometimes don't use it properly. They get in trouble in two ways: by putting their mouth on the container, releasing the gas, and freezing their tissues, or by rigging up a breathing apparatus that lets them breathe pure nitrous oxide. The problem with breathing pure nitrous oxide is that the user doesn't get oxygen, passes out, and then continues breathing only nitrous oxide until he or she is dead.

TALKING WITH KIDS ABOUT INHALANTS

• Kids need to know that these agents are very toxic and were never meant for human use. Talk about how much testing goes on for legitimate drugs and explain that when these inhalants have been tested on research animals, they make the animals very sick.

• Tell the child that any chemical he would be offered is almost certainly dangerous, either because it is toxic or because there is a real risk of getting too much and passing out. Inhalation is a dangerous way to take any drug because the agent goes directly to the brain from the lungs—it does not even pass through the liver for detoxification.

• Explain to children that they can easily die from these chemicals. The chemicals change their brain function so that their judgment is wrecked, which might make them do something really dumb like walking out in front of a car or might make them very sad and want to kill themselves.

• We strongly recommend that you explain sudden sniffing death, in the hope that it will deter kids from using these chemicals.

• It's important to teach children never to hook up any kind of breathing apparatus to allow them to inhale a drug. Explain that these devices are designed to exclude air and apply the inhalant gas through some kind of mask that covers the mouth and nose, but show them how this setup excludes oxygen from the airway. Tell them that no matter what they see on TV, all medical procedures involve mixing oxygen with the gas so that the person has enough oxygen to stay alive.

8. MARIJUANA

Marijuana use among adolescents has been declining in recent years. The University of Michigan's "Monitoring the Future" study indicates that fewer teens are trying marijuana. The number of eighth-, tenth-, and twelfth-graders who say they have tried marijuana at least once declined slightly between 1997 and 2000. The number who use marijuana regularly ("during the past month") has also declined. Although these trends are encouraging, the raw numbers show that a lot of young people still try or use marijuana. The statistics suggest that in a high school classroom with thirty students, about six may use marijuana regularly.

Marijuana use has a long and interesting history. Its use can be traced back at least as far as ancient Egypt. In the mid-1800s the use of hashish (a concentrated product of the marijuana plant) was popular among artistic and literary circles in Europe. In the United States during the early part of the twentieth century marijuana was not a very popular recreational drug. It was not until the 1950s and 1960s that marijuana came into its own as a drug of choice for a generation of young people, some of whom were searching for an altered state through which to pursue the popular ideal of "mind expansion," and some of whom were probably just looking for a recreational drug that was different from that of their parents' generation (i.e., alcohol).

As a recreational drug, marijuana presents a complicated picture. On one hand, it seems safe given its relatively low levels of toxicity and low chances of overdose. Unlike many drugs that affect the brain, including alcohol, there is no known dose of marijuana that can kill a person directly. Also, controversial, ongoing studies indicates that there is no consistent line of scientific evidence that marijuana use causes brain damage or permanent mental impairment in people. On the other hand, it has very powerful detrimental effects on learning and memory, changes the way some brain circuits process information, sticks around in the body for a long time, and can damage the lungs.

So marijuana presents a complicated picture both socially and scientifically. The points below are those that we think are the most important for young people to consider as they encounter the option to use marijuana.

THE MOST IMPORTANT THINGS TO KNOW ABOUT MARIJUANA

1. Marijuana is readily available.

Almost all adolescents report that marijuana is available at their schools or through their friends or acquaintances. One student told us that marijuana was much easier to get than alcohol because he didn't get carded when buying it. Children need to know that they will almost certainly be in environments where this drug is available. The general perception among adolescents is that marijuana is completely harmless unless you get caught with it. At some point virtually every child has to make a choice to use it or not.

Most adults would be astounded at the amount of marijuana use in our society. The Monitoring the Future survey reports that about 25 percent of high school seniors have used marijuana within the past thirty days. About 60 percent of them report having used it at some time. We believe that the increased restrictions on alcohol availability to people under 21 has helped to drive kids to use marijuana and other drugs because they can be fairly easily obtained. A young person does not have to go into a store or encounter adults to buy drugs—there is a ready supply of sellers on the street.

There is a general perception among kids (and many of their parents) that this drug is harmless. This attitude probably arises because most people know that marijuana is virtually nonlethal. Since it can't kill you, it can't be bad. That's not true, as we discuss later, but it is such a common misconception that you must bring it up when talking with kids.

Many adults used marijuana as teenagers or young adults and believe it did them no harm. They might be right. However, the marijuana they used probably contained less THC—the active ingredient—than the batches available today. In the 1960s and 1970s marijuana growing and marketing techniques had not evolved to the point they have now, and the general availability of high-potency marijuana is higher today.

2. Marijuana makes you feel good for a while.

Soon after smoking, people generally feel dreamy and relaxed. For some people this is a highly pleasant state, but there are some who simply don't like it very much. This may be in part because, although the relaxation may feel good, the accompanying impairments of mental function may be unsettling, and some people experience overt anxiety.

The subjective effects of marijuana, perhaps more than those of any other drug, are very much dependent on the individual. Generally, when one smokes a joint, there is a feeling of relaxation, melting into the surroundings, and feeling at ease with the people there. Time seems to slow down. Ideas may seem to flow more easily and take on new meaning. This often causes people to become more talkative and to interpret their conversations as more significant than they might otherwise. This mellow feeling can last for two or three hours and then slowly fades away. During this time many people also feel hungry ("the munchies").

There is a strong social connection around this drug. Since it is illegal, there's a tremendous sense of camaraderie and conspiracy in obtaining the drug, finding a place to use it, and generally avoiding detection. The social connection does not end with this clandestine activity. The flow of ideas, reduced anxiety, and shared conversation can give rise to a great sense of empathy among a group of users.

However, some people experience a down side. Marijuana almost always increases the heart rate, which may cause a sense of anxiety and, occasionally, fear or panic. The way our brains are programmed, when the heart beats faster without exercise, we interpret this as reflecting a threat. Some people have more extreme reactions and report feeling "paranoid."

3. Marijuana impairs mental functions for far longer than the feeling of being "high" lasts.

The subjective feeling of being high generally lasts a couple of hours after smoking marijuana. However, the effects of marijuana on mental functions can persist for a day or two afterward. It takes a long time for THC to be eliminated, and some of its breakdown products are also active in the brain.

Back in the 1970s, scientists at the National Institutes of Health did an interesting experiment. They injected several human volunteers with radioactive THC. They wanted to see how long it would take for the body to eliminate the THC or its active metabolites. The answer was striking—it took eight days to eliminate 90 percent of the active agents. True, much of the drug was eliminated during the first few hours after it was given, but the remainder stayed around a lot longer than expected.

Why does marijuana stay around so long? There are two reasons. First, it is very fat-soluble—that is, it is easily stored in fat after use—and then it is only slowly released from the fat over a period of many days. Second, when the body metabolizes THC, the metabolic products are also active until they are eliminated from the body through urine or feces. This is why urine tests can detect marijuana products for weeks after use.

The persistence of THC and its byproducts in the body affects mental functions as well. One study of pilots in flight simulators showed that their performance was impaired for at least twenty-four hours after smoking a modest amount of marijuana. Another study of regular marijuana users showed that their memory and problem-solving abilities were still impaired after they had abstained for at least twenty-four hours. These are the kinds of mental abilities that are critical for academic and athletic success.

4. Marijuana can cause problems in the brain and the rest of the body.

The single most important negative consequence of marijuana use is that it impairs the ability to store new information—to learn. This learning impairment lasts for beyond the euphoric effects, but it is often unrecognized by the user. Marijuana also impairs the ability of the brain to regulate physical movement by interfering with the areas that refine movements. Some frequent users become dependent on this drug and experience anxiety and sleep disturbances when they stop using it. The heart and the lungs may suffer damage from continued inhalation of smoke.

Although THC affects many parts of the brain, one of the most powerfully affected is a deeply buried region called the hippocampus. This structure is interconnected with much of the rest of the brain and is specifically wired to aid in the storage of new information. When the workings of the hippocampus are impaired, the capacity for learning is diminished. Neurobiologists can see powerful effects of THC on the brain's capacity to store information. One possibility is that THC reduces the release of the same chemical that is diminished in Alzheimer's disease (acetylcholine), and another is that it changes the way that cells within the hippocampus communicate with one another. As scientists continue to study how THC works, there is no question that it impairs learning at commonly used doses.

THC also impairs the ability of the brain to regulate physical movement. This fact is important for many reasons. Everyone knows that you should not smoke marijuana and try to drive a car. What everyone may not know is that it impairs all sorts of finely controlled and coordinated movements—like those involved in playing music and in athletic performance. So, a regular marijuana smoker may be impairing more than just his or her schoolwork or driving.

Many kids also say that marijuana reduces their anxiety, and there is every reason to believe this is true. So, what's wrong with that? Everybody wants to have less anxiety, right? Well, not necessarily. When you don't experience anxiety, you may not do what is necessary to maintain an effective life. Research shows that most kids who regularly smoke marijuana have multiple problems involving academics and other important activities. People often describe users as being "not motivated." We don't know if there is a "motivational" center in the brain, but we do know that mild anxiety is part of the motivational process.

The anxiety-reducing effects of THC, like its effects on learning, may outlast the subjective feeling of being high. So kids could experience both reduced anxiety and reduced motivation well beyond the couple of hours of feeling high. They may not even recognize that this aspect of their brain function has changed.

If kids become regular users (every day or so), a different set of concerns arises. At that point, their learning is to some extent constantly hindered, as are their normal feelings of motivation. But there's another problem. Under the constant presence of THC, the brain adapts to the drug, developing tolerance. There are natural chemicals in the brain that work like THC, and as the brain becomes less sensitive to these natural chemicals, there can be a decreased sense of well-being. When a user abruptly stops using THC, he or she may feel anxious and agitated, which tends to motivate people to continue using marijuana.

Is marijuana addictive? Well, as we just discussed, some people may feel strong withdrawal symptoms if they have been using for a while. But, as we discuss in Chapter 2 (Drug Basics), withdrawal is only a part of the addictive process. A long-lasting craving for the drug is also an important component of addiction, and we know less about this for marijuana. Many people have used this drug recreationally and have been able to stop with no problems at all. A few have become very involved with the drug and have had great difficulty giving it up.

Are adolescents more subject to addiction to marijuana? Certainly there is good evidence that exposure to some addictive substances during adolescence increases the probability of addiction to those drugs. We don't know if this is because the adolescent brain is different or because the social situation during adolescence is unique. But in any case, the earlier a child starts, the higher the probability of problems later. Whether a person is truly "addicted" to marijuana, or just has a real problem withdrawing from it, is a negligible question if the person continues to use the drug despite negative consequences.

As far as the rest of the body is concerned, the damage from marijuana is similar to that from smoking cigarettes. Marijuana smoke probably contains more toxic chemicals than cigarette smoke, but pot smokers typically do not inhale as much smoke, or smoke as many cigarettes as do regular cigarette smokers. We do know that pot smokers are more likely to experience respiratory infections and to have decreased lung function than nonsmokers. While it is not clear whether marijuana smoking alone increases the risk of lung cancer, there is some evidence that marijuana smoke changes the lung cells in ways that might lead to cancer. Likewise, smoking marijuana creates stresses on the heart from the stimulation and also the carbon monoxide contained in the smoke.

Does marijuana affect hormones and reproductive function? Here, the data are less convincing. There are reports of diminished sex drive, lower sperm counts, and male feminization, but the data are not completely convincing.

Remember that a marijuana-dependent child may have an underlying physical or mental health problem that needs professional treatment. One of us corresponded with the mother of a failing college student who was smoking a lot of marijuana. The student seemed trapped in a life of marijuana use and failure. After a complete physical workup, the student was found to have a serious problem with his thyroid function. He was trying to treat the mental symptoms of this problem by smoking pot. When a person is seriously involved with a drug, it is critical that he be fully evaluated by competent medical professionals.

TALKING WITH KIDS ABOUT MARIJUANA

• Acknowledge that marijuana is out there and that a lot of people use it—both adults and kids. This is key in developing your credibility. If you remain silent on this point, or if you take the position that only "bad" people use marijuana, kids will know you are wrong. Almost certainly a child will know someone who uses marijuana and seems to be doing just fine. We always get this question from kids: "How can Johnny smoke marijuana and get straight As if this drug is so bad?" That's the most important issue for you to confront.

• Explain that almost certainly no one has all the information about Johnny. You don't know how much marijuana he really uses (some kids lie), how potent the marijuana really is, how much he inhales, and how many problems he has apart from his academics. Most of all, you don't know what Johnny could achieve if he did not use this drug. Sometimes As are easy to come by, and a person may not realize that his performance is impaired until the competition increases or the stakes get higher. Earlier in this chapter we saw that marijuana may decrease a person's cognitive function even though it's not obvious.

• There is no getting around the fact that many kids like this drug. You cannot tell them horror stories about the few people who get panicked enough to go the emergency room, or the others who have anxiety attacks and swear never to smoke again. This just does not happen very often, and most kids wouldn't admit it if it did happen to them. A child is sure to hear from someone how good this drug makes a person feel. Your job is to understand that fact and acknowledge it, and then to explain that the good effects are offset by the possible impairments.

• Don't be afraid to talk about science. Explain that the body handles different drugs in different ways and that it handles marijuana very slowly compared to almost any other drug. Explain that the chemicals in marijuana affect the brain for as long as they are in the body—maybe for weeks.

• Explain that adolescents are in a period of life during which they need their brains to operate at full efficiency. While they may believe that the effects of the joint they smoked on Saturday night are all gone by school time on Monday morning, this is clearly not the case. Even if a kid doesn't care about academics, she still needs her brain working its best to excel in music, athletics, or even relationships with friends. Marijuana impairs the kinds of mental functions that are critical for all of these activities.

• Try to impress adolescents with the long-term consequences of their behavior. If the kid is interested in academics and is motivated to succeed, then it's important he understand the powerfully negative effects that marijuana can have on learning. Remind him that the high school and college years are a time when he'll be called on to store massive amounts of new information on a daily basis. That is much easier to do when the learning chemistry of the brain is not impaired.

• Remind him that if he smokes on the weekends and then in the middle of the week, there may be no time at which his learning and motivation are unaffected by the drug.

• If a child is not interested in school, try to find something that is important to him that involves learning or skilled movements. Is he a musician? An athlete? A skateboarder? Does he like to play complicated video games? Any of these could be markedly impaired by marijuana, and he might not want these skills impaired.

• If he seems to have lost all motivation and interest in activities that he once enjoyed, you might explain that marijuana could very well be causing this. You must remember that he is getting social support from his group of users that may be substituting for other activities. This is a difficult problem, which may be best addressed with proper counseling and medical supervision. But there are some things you can try. First, he just needs to stop using marijuana. Explain that he may well experience significant withdrawal symptoms, including anxiety, irritation, and sleeplessness, and that a physician can prescribe medicines to help him through this period. It might be the time to remind him of an old favorite activity or to start something new that is fun.

9. NICOTINE

There is a well-established laundry list of the negative health consequences of tobacco use. This is one area in which educational efforts have paid off in recent years. However, despite the best efforts of both public and private organizations to get the word out, a surprising number of children and adolescents continue to use tobacco.

Nicotine is a highly addictive drug that is legal and available in several alternative forms, including cigarettes, cigars, chewing tobacco, snuff, gum, and nicotine patches. Some of these have therapeutic benefits. For example, nicotine gum and patches can help reduce nicotine craving in addicted people, making it easier for them to quit smoking. Nicotine also enhances some mental functions, such as attention and concentration, and is being studied as a possible treatment for some cognitive problems. Medical use of nicotine is not new. Indeed, nicotine has a long history of medical use before the twentieth century, mainly because it has such powerful and obvious effects on the body.

When nicotine is delivered by gum or a skin patch with appropriate medical supervision it is relatively safe, because none of the toxic chemicals present in tobacco are present. Unfortunately, children generally don't use it in this way. They encounter it in the form of tobacco products that are both highly addictive and toxic. It's a vicious cycle—tobacco smoke damages the lungs, and oral tobacco (leaf or snuff) damages the lining of the mouth, yet both are addictive and lead to further use.

A dramatic change in attitude about smoking has taken place during the past twenty years. We have discovered and embraced scientific studies that have proven the dangers of smoking. So why do so many kids still start smoking? There are lots of reasons—advertising, hanging around with other kids who smoke, increased concentration that accompanies nicotine use, maybe even our belief that "everybody knows smoking is bad." Have we let our guard down about kids and smoking? Have we decided that "kids these days know better" or that "the schools will teach them about that"? While this may be partly true for smoking, no school-based program or antismoking advertising campaign can do the job without one-on-one follow-up. And many kids are not given any education at all about the use of oral ("smokeless") tobacco.

THE MOST IMPORTANT THINGS TO KNOW ABOUT NICOTINE

1. Nicotine is a highly addictive drug.

That nicotine is highly addictive might seem obvious when we look around at all the people who are addicted, but few people appreciate just how addictive nicotine really is. When introduced into the brain, nicotine activates the same regions within the reward system as other addictive drugs such as heroin, cocaine, and alcohol. But that's just the beginning. The way in which the nicotine reaches the brain in smokers is a set-up for addiction. Each time a smoker inhales, the blood circulating in the lungs picks up the nicotine and transports it directly to the brain—a quick, powerful hit. This kind of fast activation of the reward system is characteristic of addictive drugs. After smoking, nicotine levels in the brain fall rapidly, so it's not long before the urge to smoke returns, starting the cycle all over again.

Another factor that contributes to nicotine addiction is the development of behavioral habits that become associated with the nicotine rush in the brain. A smoker gets attached to the act of opening the pack, holding the cigarette, the feeling of lighting it, and the first drag. If a person chews or dips tobacco, the nicotine effects become associated with opening the pouch or can, packing the tobacco, spitting, and the physical feeling of having the tobacco in his mouth. These behavioral associations become part and parcel of the addiction to nicotine and can serve to maintain the addictive behavior just as the direct effects of nicotine on the brain do.

2. Nicotine may have some real value as a treatment for attention deficit hyperactivity disorder (ADHD).

Nicotine does increase a person's ability to focus and pay attention under some circumstances. If a child has some difficulty with attention and concentration, she may find that nicotine makes these things easier. Of course the problem is that most kids who use nicotine get it in the form of cigarettes, and as a "drug delivery system" this form has the disadvantages of being highly toxic to the lungs and heart as well as delivering the drug in a way that is a set-up for addiction. If you know a child who seems to have attention or concentration problems and might be using tobacco to compensate, we recommend that you have the child formally assessed for attention deficit hyperactivity disorder. Medication could be prescribed that would be more effective and much less dangerous than nicotine.

3. Smoking and depression often go hand in hand among teens.

Until recently, smoking was most often viewed as a consequence of depression, but a recent study suggests that the reverse may be true—smoking may contribute to the development of depression among teens.

Depression is a serious clinical problem among adolescents and often goes unrecognized and untreated. In fact, recent studies indicate that between 15 and 20 percent of adolescents may become depressed at some time during this developmental period —and these numbers have been on the rise. Although we've suspected a link between smoking and depression for a long time, most people thought that people started to smoke *after* they became depressed, perhaps as a means of self-medication. But a recent study involving about 15,000 teens suggests that it may be the other way around—smoking may actually lead to depression in young people.

This means that teens who smoke are at significant risk of developing depression. Obviously, it is very important to be observant about the possible effects of nicotine on mood in young people. Symptoms of depression can include consistent sadness, changes in eating or sleeping habits, and social withdrawal. It's often a complicated diagnosis, but if you have concerns about depression in a child or teen, any pediatrician's office can recommend a professional to make a formal assessment. In the process, be sure to let the doctor know if the child smokes.

4. Chewing or "dipping" tobacco *is not* a safe alternative to smoking and does not enhance athletic performance.

Many people believe that although smoking is bad, using "smokeless" tobacco is safe. Many athletes use smokeless tobacco because they think it gives them a physical edge in competition and training. Both of these beliefs are false, yet young people continue to initiate the use of these tobacco products.

A person gets about the same *peak* blood nicotine level with smokeless tobacco as by smoking a cigarette, but since the oral tobacco lasts longer it delivers a lot more nicotine, and its effects last much longer because it is absorbed more slowly. So addiction is an issue even though people don't think of smokeless tobacco products as addictive.

Long-term use of smokeless tobacco can be deadly because it significantly increases the risk of oral cancer. In addition to cancer, many diseases of the mouth occur in chronic users of smokeless tobacco. For example, users have nearly two and a half times as many dental cavities as nonusers, in part because both leaf and plug tobacco preparations contain about 20 to 35 percent sugar. Recession of the gums is also common with chronic use, often leading to periodontal disease, which can result in the loss of teeth or bone. One study found that among high school students, about three hours use per day, on average, caused an increase in these diseases. Another study found diseases of the delicate inner lining of the cheeks and mouth in 49 percent of high school users. One particularly dangerous lesion common to the mouths of smokeless tobacco users is called *leukoplakia*. This lesion is identified as a white patch or plaque and can be precancerous.

So why do people use these products? In part because they really do have some effects on alertness and mental function. People appear to be a little better able to concentrate their attention on certain kinds of mental tasks while using smokeless tobacco. Some studies have shown scores on tests of concentration and timed mental arithmetic to be slightly higher in people using smokeless tobacco. However, these improvements, even when present, are slight and certainly not worth the risk of addiction and other health effects of using the drug.

Lots of people start using smokeless tobacco because they are athletes and have been told that it will enhance their reaction time, strength, or visual tracking ability. It has none of these effects. Well-controlled studies of athletes have shown no positive effects on any of these measures relating to athletic performance. But there are some negative effects on exercise and athletic performance that young athletes should know about. Smokeless tobacco has actually been shown to *decrease* the speed and force of leg movements during reaction-time tests. It also has negative effects on the heart during exercise—increasing heart rate and decreasing the output of blood from the heart during physically demanding exercise. And during moderate exercise, smokeless tobacco appears to increase the build-up of lactate in the blood, possibly increasing muscle fatigue and decreasing endurance.

TALKING WITH KIDS ABOUT NICOTINE

• First, let children know that just because a drug is legal for use by adults does not mean it's safe. You can compare nicotine to alcohol and point out that alcohol is legal for adults, but that many adults become addicted to it—just like nicotine. Laws are good and help people to know what's right and wrong, but they are not always consistent, and legality doesn't imply safety.

• Explain that the drug nicotine is in all tobacco products—not just cigarettes—and nicotine can change the brain in ways that make it very hard to stop using the drug.

• Point out that, unlike some other addictive drugs, nicotine does not produce a distinct feeling of being buzzed or high, which means that the addiction can creep up on the user. People tend to think of drugs as addictive only if they produce a strong change in the way they feel. But nicotine is unusual in this way—it's highly addictive without causing the user to feel very different.

• Talk about the fact that addiction to nicotine involves the development of complex habits—the brain changes to create a physical need for the drug, but the behavioral habits associated with its use are also powerful components of the addiction. Talk about how hard it is to break habits. If the child plays sports you may be able to identify a habit that he is working to break in order to get better—not dropping the back elbow before swinging a baseball bat, stutter-stepping before kicking a soccer ball, always going to the right off the dribble. Point out that once these bad habits are established, it's very hard to change them. The little things that people do along with smoking or dipping tobacco are similarly hard habits to break and can add to the brain changes that keep people hooked on nicotine for life.

• Remind the teen that her brain runs on chemical signals, which regulate both thinking and feelings. Point out that sometimes those chemical signals can go wrong, and feelings can sink into a consistent state of unhappiness that may reflect a medical problem called depression. Let her know that nicotine is a powerful drug that affects this brain chemistry, and it looks like one of those effects in teens may be to tilt the brain chemistry toward depression.

• In general, when dealing with a teen who might be depressed, it's important to remember she might not be able or willing to articulate her feelings. She may simply be too depressed and/or frightened to open up easily. Under these circumstances you can assure her that you are there and will help. Getting proper medical evaluation and treatment—which certainly should include a quit-smoking program if necessary—is the first step. But it takes consistent support and involvement to see a person through a depressive episode.

• Make it clear that there is a lot of misinformation about smoke-less tobacco. Kids may hear that it's "safe because it's not as bad as smoking," but this is absolutely not true. Point out that one reason the lungs are so easily damaged by cigarette smoke is because of their very sensitive linings. Lungs let us know that smoke is bad by causing us to cough. The lining of the mouth is also very sensitive, and when tobacco is placed there we also get a similar signal—a strong tingling and slight burning sensation.

• If the child you're talking with is an athlete, let him know that despite what he might hear, tobacco will not improve his physical performance. Smokeless tobacco releases a lot of nicotine into the bloodstream, which makes the heart beat faster but less efficiently during exercise. Not only that, but the nicotine may make muscles become tired sooner than they would normally, thus limiting endurance in sports.

10. OPIATES AND SEDATIVES

There are a great many drugs within the categories of opiates and sedatives, but we have placed them together in one chapter because their bottom-line dangers are quite similar—they powerfully suppress brain activity and can result in death from a single high dose. The *opiates*—such as morphine, which is used as a medicine to control pain, and heroin, which is abused for its euphoric effects—work by activating some very specific kinds of receptors in the brain. These receptors are present for good reason—to control our perception of pain so that we can survive under traumatic circumstances—and the brain makes its own opiates to activate these receptors when necessary. But the brain knows exactly how much of these natural opiates to use, and when, and uses them very sparingly. People who use opiates recreationally often administer much more than the brain would release even under the most extreme circumstances. This can cause an incredibly pleasant "rush" of good feeling and relaxation that many compare to orgasm, which is part of the reason it's so easy to get addicted to these drugs. The problem is that if too much is taken, the centers in the brain that keep us breathing can shut down, resulting in death.

Sedatives include barbiturates such as phenobarbital and pentobarbital (Nembutal), chloral hydrate, benzodiazepines (such as Valium and Ativan), and methaqualone (Quaaludes). These drugs don't act by stimulating opiate receptors, and they are not as addictive as some opiates, but they do affect brain regions that control vital functions such as alertness, learning, motor coordination, and breathing. A person on one of these drugs is physically slowed down and cognitively impaired. At high doses people can appear semiconscious. *As with opiates, the most pressing danger is an acute overdose, which can kill.* But sedatives also severely impair movement and coordination, so that a person who has taken them is much more liable to have serious accidents.

THE MOST IMPORTANT THINGS TO KNOW ABOUT OPIATES AND SEDATIVES

1. Opiates are highly addictive drugs.

Since recreational doses of opiates stimulate the brain's natural opiate receptors so powerfully, and because the feeling that the user gets is so pleasant, the process of addiction occurs very rapidly with these drugs. Addiction is a complicated process involving changes in both the brain and behavior of the individual. Opiates affect both of these. The system of brain receptors they stimulate can change rapidly, adapting to the presence of the drug so that when it is not around the person feels the need to replenish the supply. In addition, the initial rush of feeling associated with the drug is so pleasant that some people come to crave it to the point that they will do almost anything to reexperience the high.

2. Opiate addiction is a serious medical problem.

This is a simple point, but one that is sometimes not understood. People can get off of opiates, but it is critical that the effort take place under medical and psychological supervision. The brain has to recover and readapt to not having the drug around. The person also must adapt to significant changes in lifestyle. Medicines are available that can make the process a bit easier, and in combination with psychological help and social support these can stack the deck for recovery in favor of the patient.

3. Opiates can kill with one high dose, and it's impossible to know the potency or purity of street drugs.

This is the most dangerous aspect of opiate use. There have been many tragic cases of people buying drugs on the street and dying from overdose after taking what they think is their usual "safe" dosage.

4. Some nonopiate sedatives can kill with one high dose, while others are safer. But they all are particularly dangerous when combined with opiates or other sedative drugs.

Sedatives are the drugs that users call "downers." These include benzodiazepines such as Valium, Librium, and Ativan, along with barbiturates such as pentobarbital (Nembutal) and phenobarbital. They are different from opiates and produce effects somewhat like alcohol. This makes sense because they work on the same GABA system that we talked about in the chapter on alcohol (Chapter 4). The sedative drugs produce very different effects at low and high doses. At low doses they cause a sense of relaxation and relief of anxiety, as well as a generally "mellowed" feeling. (This is different from the opiate high, in that the sedatives do not produce the extreme rush of pleasure that the opiates do.) At higher doses people begin to feel lightheaded and dizzy. They might become quite drowsy and uncoordinated and begin to slur their speech. These symptoms are not too different from when a person gets drunk. In fact, one problem is that people sometimes take sedatives along with alcohol or other depressant drugs in order to enhance the effects. This can be really dangerous because the effects of the drugs on breathing and movement combine as well, and can quickly move a person dangerously close to an overdose. Overdose deaths from sedatives alone are pretty rare, but all bets are off when they are combined with other depressant drugs.

TALKING WITH KIDS ABOUT OPIATES AND SEDATIVES

• Explain that some drugs can cause the brain to change in ways that cause the person to feel sick when the drug is not present. For a younger child you can use the example of receiving a treat on a regular basis. The first time you surprise him by spontaneously taking him to a movie or giving him some candy, it feels very special and good. But if you give him the treat every day after school, and then abruptly stop, he'll miss it and maybe even feel angry that it is missing. Tell him that those feelings are very mild compared to the bad feelings that can occur when a person takes opiates for a little while and then stops. In this case he will feel very sick and be desperate for the drug.

• For older children, point out that opiate drugs make people feel very good at first, and many people say the first few times they use opiates are the best feelings they have ever had. This effect is so powerful that one person we know actually broke

117

down and cried after she had received an opiate drug to help with pain after a medical procedure. She felt desperately sad that she could not live every moment with that feeling of pleasure and well-being. Fortunately, she knew enough to avoid taking the drug on her own because she understood that the intense feeling of pleasure would diminish over time and that she would come to crave more and more of the drug.

• Explain that opiate drugs have legitimate medical uses and that medical doses are calculated very carefully to ensure that people are not hurt by taking too much.

• Point out that when opiates are used as medicine for pain, the drug is very pure so doctors know the doses can be carefully calculated. Also, the person giving the drug is always careful to give only as much as is needed to control the person's pain. This is because at higher doses the effects can be dangerous.

• When talking with young children, it's important not to tell them things that are too frightening or easily misunderstood. Using analogies like "It will make you go to sleep and never wake up" might seem clear and easy to understand, but has the potential to make a child terrified of falling asleep. We think it's better to explain that the child's brain helps keep her alive and that these particular drugs can make the brain stop working.

• The issues of potency and purity are more relevant for older children, who are more likely to encounter an offer to try opiates. It is important to emphasize how powerful these chemicals are and how critical are the brain functions they affect. Next, point out that they have no control whatsoever over what is in a sample of a drug that might be offered. It's impossible to judge purity with the naked eye, or even to tell the difference between any number of drugs that may have the appearance of opiates as a white or brown powder. Opiates in pill form that have been diverted from legitimate medical use can be dangerous as well. The risk of overdose is just as real. The user won't know the proper dosage, or probably even what the drug really is.

• Since many sedatives come in pill form and are obviously produced as medicines, the old lesson that medicines are only safely taken as prescribed by a physician comes in handy here—particularly if the child has been taught it from an early age.

• Point out that sometimes when drugs that have similar actions are combined, the effects can be much more powerful than either drug alone. Indeed, in some instances it can be greater than a simple additive effect. Emphasize that alcohol is a kind of drug that can have dangerous effects on its own (see the Alcohol chapter) and that sedatives have some of the same kinds of effects. When combined, alcohol and sedatives can cause severe memory impairment, unconsciousness, and even death.

• Increased awareness about drunk driving and better enforcement of drunk driving laws has led some to think that if they drink less, they can take sedatives to get "drunker" and still be safe to drive. This is completely wrong. In fact, a person with both sedatives and alcohol in their system is even more dangerous on the road than a person high on one or the other alone.

11. ECSTASY, GHB, AND KETAMINE: THE SO-CALLED PARTY DRUGS

The group of drugs that includes Ecstasy, GHB, and ketamine are well named as "party drugs" or "club drugs" because they have become popular as part of the social scene from teenage raves to sophisticated urban thirty-something parties. Ecstasy, in particular, is achieving virtually epidemic popularity among teenagers, and is the only illegal drug gaining in usage among kids.

Ecstasy is a chemical called MDMA (methylenedioxymethamphetamine), which, as you can see from the chemical name, is a cousin of amphetamine. Ecstasy produces effects unlike any other known drug—a profound sense of peace, love, and empathy. It was invented early in the twentieth century, but lay dormant until the 1970s when some psychotherapists and pharmacologists hoped that it might be helpful to people in understanding themselves and their relationships with others. It slowly became a "legal" recreational drug that was popular at a few colleges and among people committed to using drugs for personal insight. In 1985, the government decided it was too toxic for medical use and made it illegal. Still, that did not stop it from becoming popular, particularly with teenagers.

GHB (gamma hydroxybutyric acid) is a sedative drug that is used as an anesthetic agent and treatment for alcoholism in Europe. It is a naturally occurring chemical in the human brain, and nerve cells in many parts of the brain have sensors for it. We don't understand exactly what it does in the brain except make people sleep. At low doses, there is a mild euphoria and release from anxiety like that produced by alcohol, and at higher levels, there are similar feelings to being really drunk. The first recreational users were body builders, who believed that it would make them stronger (research has not confirmed this). People found that GHB could be easily synthesized, and its popularity grew as recipes were published on the internet.

Ketamine (Special K) is another anesthetic drug, which is legally produced in the United States. We talked about this drug in the chapter on hallucinogens (Chapter 6). It works in an unusual way and does not put people into as deep a sleep. It's used mostly for animals and children, because adult humans tend to have frightening hallucinations from it. Teenagers like it for its alcohol-like buzz, and some enjoy a feeling of being outside themselves, so it's become a moderately popular recreational drug.

THE MOST IMPORTANT THINGS TO KNOW
ABOUT ECSTASY

1. Ecstasy works by releasing massive amounts of the chemical serotonin in the brain, which makes the user feel very good.

Serotonin is a brain chemical that regulates many brain processes, including appetite, sleep, body temperature, memory, and sense of well-being. Releasing large amounts of serotonin quickly produces powerful psychological effects.

You've heard about serotonin before if you're familiar with antidepressant drugs. Prozac, Paxil, and many other antidepressants are called selective serotonin reuptake inhibitors or SSRIs. When nerve cells containing serotonin get a signal from other cells, they release serotonin into the brain. To conserve the chemical and to limit its time of action, they actively recycle it back in. The SSRIs work by preventing nerve cells from recycling some of the serotonin they release. A depressed person feels better when there is a little more serotonin in his brain, and his sleep, appetite, and sense of well-being are improved.

Ecstasy works differently than the SSRIs, because it enters the nerve cells and causes them to spill large amounts of their serotonin whether they have a signal to do so or not. So the user experiences a marked improvement in mood. She feels euphoria, a loss of anxiety, peace, tranquility, and empathy and love for others. People say that their sense of touch is enhanced, so they enjoy experimenting with different textures. One of Dr. Wilson's daughters went to a "rave" (an all-night party with dancing to loud music and open drug use) where there was a lot of Ecstasy use and came home describing it as such a loving, peaceful, and caring environment that she wanted to be told again "exactly what was wrong with using this drug."

Here is another opportunity for parental supervision to play a role in protecting kids. Know where your kids are going and what will be in that environment. If kids are going to all-night raves, it's a safe bet that drugs will be there. If you have any questions, ask your local police department.

2. The first use of Ecstasy can be injurious or fatal.

The massive release of serotonin can raise body temperature and cause serious problems. Ecstasy is often used in hot dance environments where there is a lot of physical activity. Remember that Ecstasy is a stimulant cousin of amphetamine, and like all stimulants it makes people want to move around. So dancing is a natural outlet, and users tend to get hot. The serotonin the drug releases disrupts the ability of the body to regulate its temperature, which can cause seizures and brain injury. Another problem is that people drink so much water while trying to stay cool that the concentration of sodium in their body is reduced to the point where the heart and brain no longer function properly. The increased heat and seizures may cause breakdown of muscle tissue and the release of lots of chemicals from the muscle. Finally, the blood tends to coagulate and stop up the veins, leading to death.

3. People feel bad after the effects of Ecstasy wear off.

Because Ecstasy releases so much serotonin, the brain has less of it to use for a few days after Ecstasy use. This makes people feel bad for those days. The serotonin spilled by Ecstasy has to be replaced by the nerve cells and this takes time. While the serotonin level is low, the user feels depressed—he's dysphoric (just feels crummy), has a poor appetite, sleeps poorly, and is anxious. Recovery can take a few days. If the person is naturally depressed, this is an especially risky time. Remember that depression can be a deadly disorder because depressed people may attempt suicide. The combination of background depression plus the depression from Ecstasy withdrawal can be a real problem.

4. The latest medical research shows that repeated use of Ecstasy damages serotonin-containing nerve cells.

Damage to serotonin-containing nerve cells is the most serious aspect of Ecstasy. The best medical research in both animal and human studies is showing that Ecstasy is a neurotoxin. Repeated use kills the parts of nerve cells that release serotonin, and we don't know when or if recovery occurs.

This is not only the worst aspect of Ecstasy, it is the most controversial. Frankly, lots of recreational users just love Ecstasy, and they strongly resist any message that it is toxic. Also, there is a group of scientists and clinicians who believe it should be made available for clinical use with individuals. They too tend to dismiss any studies that show the drug is toxic. They argue that it is safe in low doses. *The problem is that we don't know how low a dose is low enough.*

Animal research shows that repeated dosing at levels corresponding to human use damages the serotonin system, and recovery may never occur. Rats have been studied for one year and primates for seven years after repeated exposure to Ecstasy, and their brains have not fully recovered. Research studies cannot detect small amounts of damage, so we don't know whether this damage occurs with the first use.

Research with human Ecstasy users also points to real problems. Brain imaging studies of the serotonin systems of long-term users shows lasting impairment. Psychological exams show that long-term users have memory problems as well. Young humans (and animals) probably have an excess of serotonin function, so damage might not be noticeable right away. However, people probably lose serotonin function as they age, so those who have inflicted damage to this system in their youth may have a tendency to become depressed in later years.

TALKING WITH KIDS ABOUT ECSTASY

• Point out that Ecstasy is a very powerful chemical that enters the brain and releases a massive amount of the brain's natural chemical serotonin. For younger kids, you can use the analogy of the gas grill. The gas jets in the grill release small, steady amounts of gas so that the flame is well contained. But if a large amount of gas is released all at once, there is an explosion, as an uncontrolled fire.

• Acknowledge that people say Ecstasy makes a person feel full of love and empathy for the few hours it's in the body. There is no sense in trying to downplay this aspect of Ecstasy, because you will be lying, and kids will know it. But this feeling is not only transient, it allows a person to make bad decisions, so he or she fails to avoid dangerous situations—whether riding with a drunk driver, trying other drugs and combinations of drugs, or having unsafe sex. After all, humans feel fear and caution for a reason, and being at a party where there are a lot of drugs puts a person at risk.

• This is a great time to make the point that almost all drugs do more than just one thing. Sure, Ecstasy makes you feel good, but because it can alter other body processes it can be dangerous. Also, how does a person know how much she is getting? Ecstasy is not a legally manufactured pill—all of it comes from illicit labs, so it's not possible to know how much is in one dose.

• Don't let kids be misled by outfits that test pills to be sure they are Ecstasy. They cannot screen for everything, and they cannot determine how much Ecstasy is in the pill. Moreover, Ecstasy itself can be dangerous, even if it is pure.

• *Water intoxication* is something that all kids need to know about. When anyone drinks too much water, he dilutes the amount of sodium in the blood, which causes disruption of electrical activity in all parts of the body. That's why athletes drink fluids containing sodium on hot days when they are sweating a lot. A number of Ecstasy deaths have resulted from kids *intentionally* drinking lots of water, thinking that they can prevent the toxicity.

• Remind kids that for almost all psychoactive drugs there is a period of recovery after the drug is used—for example, a hangover from alcohol. For serotonin, you might use an example of a slowly filling container. If it tips over and spills its contents, time is required for it to refill.

• Many kids become depressed at some time in their adolescence, and this is a good time to talk about that subject. Have kids talk about what it feels like to be depressed and how miserable it is. Then remind them that Ecstasy leaves people feeling this way.

• By all means teach kids to tell someone if they are really depressed. The suicidal tendency that comes with depression often is out of the depressed person's control and can only be stopped with help from other people. Help kids to know that they can talk about these feelings.

• Kids just don't have the ability to easily project current behavior into future consequences, so arguing that they may become depressed or forgetful in the future may not work. Even more than for smoking, there is a big disconnect between how good they feel on the drug and bad consequences far off in the future. But they need to be told. Try to make the analogy to pruning a tree. Using Ecstasy is like trimming off the ends of the branches. It may not be very noticeable at first, but with time, the shape of the tree really changes.

• What happens when a branch is pruned? The tree continues to grow, but in a different pattern. It puts out sprouts all around the pruned area, trying to reestablish a branch. That's what the brain does when it has been affected by Ecstasy. When the serotonin-releasing parts of the cells are killed by Ecstasy, some of the cells die, but some branch out trying to get back to normal. The problem is that the new branches are not exactly like the original ones. Likewise, the regrowing serotonin neurons probably apply serotonin to places it should not be in the brain. This may cause as many problems as the loss of serotonin itself.

• No matter what kids hear, scientists just don't know if any use of Ecstasy is safe.

THE MOST IMPORTANT THINGS TO KNOW ABOUT GHB

1. GHB is a drug that induces sleep, and it can kill, especially when taken in combination with alcohol.

GHB sedates the central nervous system, including the parts of the brain that tell us to keep breathing. Alcohol can make this effect even more powerful. Overdose with GHB causes people to stop breathing. You breathe because your brain senses the need for oxygen and sends the signals out to your muscles to fill your lungs. Sedative drugs are designed to make people go to sleep without suppressing their breathing, but they are not perfect—most of them will suppress breathing in high doses, and that's the way they kill. GHB is a colorless and tasteless liquid that is often mixed with alcoholic drinks; its presence is undetectable. Since alcohol is also a sedative, the combination can be deadly.

GHB also produces profound amnesia for the time a person

is intoxicated with it. Because of this quality and the ability to mask it in a drink, it is used as a date-rape drug.

2. Repeated use of GHB causes powerful withdrawal symptoms.

The brain adapts to repeated use of GHB over a period of months, and withdrawal can be so severe that hospitalization is required.

GHB use started with the body-building community. A scientific paper was published showing that GHB released growth hormone in the body, and body-builders decided they would use it to increase their muscle mass. Nobody ever proved it can make a person stronger, but people kept using the drug anyway. Now we are seeing people who use it regularly become so dependent that they must take the drug every two to four hours. If they stop, they go into withdrawal and can't sleep or function effectively. Within twenty-four hours of withdrawal, some of these users become psychotic and have to be put in a hospital where they are heavily drugged and placed in restraints. Psychiatrists tell us it is the worst type of drug withdrawal they have seen.

3. Other chemicals convert to GHB in the body.

Because GHB is a naturally occurring chemical in the body, the body is capable of manufacturing it from other chemicals. Two of these chemicals, GBL (gamma butyrolactone) and 4-BD (4-amino butyrodione), are made into GHB in the brain. Recent laws have restricted the sale and manufacture of GHB, and some control GBL. However, 4-BD is a solvent that is readily available, and it is just as effective as GHB. It's being sold under various labels as a body-building product. So the government restriction is doing little to suppress the availability of GHB-like chemicals. Stress to kids that any of these products can lead to the same problems as

GHB—lethal overdose, amnesia and date rape, and withdrawal problems.

TALKING WITH KIDS ABOUT GHB

• Tell kids that GHB can kill by sedating a person so heavily that they stop breathing. Most important, tell them that mixing this drug with alcohol makes it more deadly.

• GHB is used as a date-rape drug because it can be added to a drink without a person knowing it's there. Tell children that they should not accept drinks without being very careful about what might be in the drink.

• Most important, warn kids that if they ever drink something and feel different than they expect to feel—for example, more intoxicated than they might from a single drink of alcohol—they should get help. GHB could have been in the cocktail. (This is quite common in party environments and has happened to friends of our daughters.)

• Explain to kids that when GHB is used regularly, the brain changes to adapt to it. These changes make the brain "need" GHB to function properly, because the brain is adapting to the large amount of GHB the person is taking rather than depending on its own supply. Thus, when people try to give it up after using it a while, they have major problems.

• Especially warn kids about buying products at the gym. Great amounts of GHB and chemicals like it are distributed at gyms, supposedly for body-building purposes. The chemicals do nothing for building bodies and do a lot for trashing brains.

THE MOST IMPORTANT THING TO KNOW ABOUT KETAMINE

Ketamine is an anesthetic that causes the brain to ignore pain. Like other anesthetics, it can kill at high doses.

Ketamine works by causing the brain to disassociate pain signals from a feeling of distress, so that a person ignores any pain. However, this dissociation produces hallucinations at clinical levels. In high doses it can kill, like other sedatives.

This drug is primarily used only for kids and animals because adults wake up and have hallucinations. Young children don't seem to have this problem when the drug is used as a medicine, which is another example of the differences between the adult and child brain. Teenagers must be somewhere in between, because many of them experience the hallucinations and like the feeling that ketamine produces. Ketamine can kill either children or adults if they take too much.

TALKING WITH KIDS ABOUT KETAMINE

• Teach kids that ketamine is a sedative like others and that it kills in high doses. However, because very few deaths from the drug have been reported, it is unlikely your children will have heard of anyone's getting into trouble.

• The greatest risk with ketamine is the same as that for other hallucinogens—that a person will do something stupid while under the influence of the drug. Caution children that ketamine is like other hallucinogens and that they may make very unsafe decisions while under its influence.

12. STEROIDS AND OTHER PERFORMANCE-ENHANCING DRUGS

Performance-enhancing drugs are all those chemicals that are supposed to make us bigger, thinner, faster, steadier, or stronger. They are all the rage now that athletes at the highest competitive levels are using and abusing them. You see them everywhere—the supermarket shelves, the nutrition stores, on the internet, and in the gym. Everybody wants to find a supplement to make them better in some way or another. So what's the truth about these drugs, and what do you tell kids?

If you look at the number of different product names, you could be overwhelmed. In fact, there are a lot of products, and the area is so complicated that we wrote an entire book about it: *Pumped: Straight Facts for Athletes About Drugs, Supplements, and Training* (W. W. Norton, 2000). In this section we only discuss steroids (diet aids are covered in Chapter 13, Stimulants). Steroids are the most problematic performance-enhancing drugs and the only ones for which we have information in developing humans. Still, for all of these chemicals, we can give you the bottom line right now: *Our position is that children with growing brains and bodies should avoid the use of every one of these compounds.* We don't know enough about the effects of any of these agents on the growing human to say that they are safe, and in fact we know some of them are dangerous.

THE MOST IMPORTANT THINGS TO KNOW ABOUT STEROIDS

1. Not all steroids are the same.

There are two kinds of steroids that you hear about: *catabolic steroids* and *anabolic steroids*. The catabolic ones are prescribed by doctors to suppress inflammatory processes and to help with asthma, while the anabolic steroids, like testosterone, build muscle. The difference between steroid types is often a source of confusion and concern. Catabolic steroids not only suppress inflammation, but they actually break down muscle. It's the anabolic steroids that people use to promote muscle growth. Testosterone is the best-known anabolic agent, and most anabolic drugs athletes use increase testosterone or provide extra amounts of it by one method or another.

2. Anabolic steroids can have powerful effects on development of the body.

Testosterone is a sex hormone. It is one of the main factors that differentiate men from women, and it is critical to how our bodies and brains develop. Men have much more testosterone than women, and that's why they have deeper voices, more body hair, and bigger muscles. The surge in testosterone that occurs at puberty is why boys grow so fast and change so much in such a short period of time. Development normally depends on getting the right amount of testosterone at the right time. Supplementing testosterone levels during development can have disastrous effects. It can so confuse the body's internal signaling systems that boys may stop growing and girls may develop male characteristics.

3. The normal, fully developed male has enough testosterone.

Men make all the testosterone their body needs. This is a big secret that supplement manufacturers don't talk about. Men have enough testosterone to saturate all of their testosterone sensors. To get any additional effect, body-builders have to raise their testosterone levels by a huge amount—100 to 10,000 times normal. We don't know why this enormous boost in testosterone builds muscle, but we think it might be because, at these levels, the anabolic steroids block the actions of the catabolic steroids, which break down muscle. However, at these levels, there are definite negative health effects, including heart and liver problems.

Over-the-counter anabolic supplements do not produce these kinds of testosterone levels. Some of these chemicals increase testosterone a little, but not enough to make any difference, while others may actually increase estrogen. What boy wants to have more estrogen running around in his body? Probably not the kid who is thinking about building muscle.

4. The claims of supplement manufacturers are not regulated by the government.

A 1994 law made supplements more accessible in the United States by removing much of the regulatory power of the Food

133

and Drug Administration. Thus, marketers can make claims without having to back them up with rigorous research.

Very few people know what happened in 1994. In that year Congress passed a law that treats "natural" compounds quite differently than drugs made by the pharmaceutical industry. For the drugs your doctor prescribes, the manufacturer must prove to the FDA that the drugs are both safe and effective. The same is not true for supplements made from natural compounds—the manufacturer can claim anything, and the burden is on the FDA to prove otherwise. Given the limited resources of the FDA and the vast number of supplements, it is impossible for the agency to patrol them effectively. The net result is that lots of supplements are sold by claims that are not well substantiated by legitimate medical research.

TALKING WITH KIDS ABOUT STEROIDS

• Make sure that kids understand that taking catabolic steroids for asthma or some other problem is not the same as abusing testosterone-generating compounds. Kids who are taking steroids for their asthma are taking medicine, not illegal supplements, and they should not stop. Using steroids for asthma doesn't build muscle, and catabolic steroids won't disqualify an athlete from a sports event.

• Kids need to know that naturally occurring testosterone controls very important characteristics of the growth of their bodies. Almost all kids have the right amount at the right time, and adding extra is like putting too much fertilizer on a plant—it either stops growth and kills the plant or makes it into something abnormal.

• Girls should be strongly warned that adding testosterone at any point in their lives, but especially during growth, can give them the characteristics of boys. They can grow unwanted body hair, develop deeper voices, or even have distorted genitalia (enhanced growth of the clitoris).

• Brain development also depends on sex hormones, and it's fair to tell kids we don't know too much about this yet. However, it's just not wise to take the chance that something as important as brain function be put at risk by using these chemicals.

• Warn children that while their bodies are still developing, over-the-counter supplements may be able to raise testosterone enough to change their development. We just don't have the research data yet, and it's not worth taking the chance.

• Explain to kids that those huge guys they see had to take testosterone or other powerful drugs that produce it in the body. These drugs are not available as over-the-counter supplements and are illegal for use without a prescription.

• Find a drugstore with a good and friendly pharmacist who is willing to talk with your child about this topic. Have the pharmacist explain just how careful drug companies have to be with a prescribed drug compared to companies that sell supplements. We think it's a worthwhile exercise that will make a big impression. If you can't do that, walk your child through the drugstore and make the point yourself.

13. STIMULANTS: FROM REWARD TO ADDICTION— THE GOOD AND THE BAD

When you hear the word *stimulant*, you probably think of drugs that promote talking, moving, staying awake, and even thinking a bit better—like a good cup of coffee. But the stimulants we discuss in this chapter do much more than just "get you going." They interact with a very specific part of the brain called the "reward system," and it is through their actions in that neural network that some of them are extraordinarily addictive.

Some of the drugs we talk about are the hard-core drugs that you hear a lot about in the news, such as cocaine and methamphetamine. But later in the chapter we describe stimulants that can be medically useful, such as Ritalin (methylphenidate) and drugs in diet aids like ephedrine. The key to understanding all of these stimulant drugs lies in understanding the brain's reward system, so we deal with that first.

The Brain's Reward System

One of the most important parts of the brain, and one that most people don't even know exists, is the reward system. This is a network of several groups of nerve cells that work together to make humans (and animals) do what is good for preservation of the species—activities like finding food and water, having sex, winning battles, and having good social interactions. We certainly don't know everything about how this network of nerve cells works, but we know enough to understand why stimulants do what they do.

The first activity of the reward system is to make us *pay attention* to something that meets our needs for preservation of the species. The scientists who study this subject use the word *salience* (or meaning) to describe how the reward changes the way we respond to a particular cue. Let's use the example of grandmother's chocolate cake.

Your reward system has associated eating your grandmother's cake with great pleasure and satisfaction because fat and sugar stimulate the reward system. So your reward system has associated "cues" with her cake. You start looking forward to that cake when you turn the corner to her house and as you drive in the driveway. You have learned to pay attention to the stimuli in the environment that signal "cake is on the way." Once you get out of the car, you *focus* on that cake. That's the second thing the reward system does—it helps you focus on the task. Then you head straight for the kitchen. The reward system facilitates *purposeful movement*. Attention, focus, and movement, these are the tools that the reward system give us to fulfill our basic needs.

What's interesting about the reward system is that you don't really have to have an immediate or urgent need for it to function. Your reward system has associated eating your grandmother's chocolate cake with great pleasure and satisfaction. So even if you're not particularly hungry, when you see one of those wonderful cakes, you probably begin to salivate and think of having a slice right away. You might even begin to obsess about how to convince your grandmother to cut that cake before dinner.

We can illustrate one other characteristic of the reward system with grandmother's cake, and that's its dependence on a degree of *novelty*. You know that if you have full access to that wonderful cake every day, eventually you would get tired of it and it would lose its attractiveness. If your grandmother switched to an equally delicious coconut cake, you'd get worked up all over again. The novelty requirement of the reward system ensures that you select a variety of delicious foods and not just stick to one.

All of these characteristics of the reward system have great value in survival of the species. It doesn't take much thought to understand how the reward system might function in sex, or game playing, or any of myriad activities. In fact, almost everything we do, we do because it is in some way "rewarding" or on the way to meeting a reward-system need. We work to get money to buy food and other things we want. We seek novel experiences like travel, new friends, or new games. The human brain is so complex that it is capable of making all sorts of associations and connections of cues and experiences back to the reward circuits, which leads it to enact very complex behaviors to satisfy our reward drives.

The next step is to understand just a little about the brain chemistry that powers the reward system. The key element is the neurochemical *dopamine*. Based on years of medical research, we now believe that dopamine is a key player in the function of these circuits. Brain imaging studies of animals and humans show the release of dopamine by reward-system nerve cells whenever the animal or person detects a cue associated with reward. That cue could be a picture of grandmother's chocolate cake, an attractive sex partner, or a pile of money. A cue to anything that is meaningful in the reward system releases dopamine and begins the process of trying to get it.

Now to talk about drugs, one central point is key: *All addictive drugs release the chemical dopamine in the brain's reward system.* These drugs get right into the heart of the brain's reward system and elevate the level of one of its key chemicals. No matter what the chemical or the activity, if you're addicted to it, it's partly because your brain gets a blast of dopamine when you get a cue to that activity. That release of dopamine makes you feel good and you want more, whether it's nicotine that releases just a touch of dopamine with each cigarette, or cocaine that releases lots of dopamine. Cocaine produces all the characteristics of stimulating the reward system—only a lot stronger. Your heart rate and breathing increase. There is a tendency to move around and talk more. You become euphoric and remember the experience as just wonderful. And it is wonderful, because the drug tapped into the very basis of the reward system.

How Does Addiction Develop?

Here's how you become addicted. Your brain remembers the absolutely wonderful experience you had with that line of cocaine. It makes you pay attention to all the aspects of the cocaine experience by storing all sorts of cues associated with it—the person that gave it to you, the room you were in, the texture and appearance of the drug, and an array of other perceptions. So the next time you detect any of those cues, your reward system makes you pay attention—even the cues trigger release of dopamine. Your heart rate increases and you get excited and motivated to get some cocaine. Yet, at this point you're not completely down the path to addiction.

The latest research shows that addiction can be a slow

process. Animal experiments show that just a few exposures to a drug don't make an addict. It takes multiple exposures over a prolonged period—maybe weeks to months. Over this time some important chemical changes occur in the brain that make the individual constantly crave the drug. We really don't yet know all about these changes, but we know they occur. When they do, it can be very difficult to stop using the drug. Even prolonged periods of abstinence don't necessarily correct the problem, and people remain sensitive to reinitiating the drug for years after they have stopped.

Just as all addictive drugs stimulate the reward system, so do addictive behaviors, like compulsive sex, overeating, or even gambling. Anything that a human finds rewarding can become an addiction if it is excessively pursued. We don't know why different people are sensitive to becoming addicted to different drugs or activities, but it's probably based in the variations in individual chemistry. Perhaps some drugs or activities release more dopamine in one person than another.

THE MOST IMPORTANT THINGS TO KNOW ABOUT STIMULANTS

1. A variety of chemicals are stimulants, and some of them easily produce addiction, while others don't.

Cocaine, crack cocaine, methamphetamine, and crystal methamphetamine are powerful stimulants that are highly addictive. Ritalin (methylphenidate) and other drugs taken orally are also stimulants. They can be safe if taken according to a doctor's orders, but they can be addictive if taken in excess.

It is important to recognize that huge differences exist in the spectrum of stimulant drugs. The ones that are most addictive are the ones that produce the "buzz" or euphoria. The brain becomes euphoric with *rapid* increases in dopamine, which happens when the drug gets to the brain quickly. Snorted cocaine, smoked crack cocaine, and smoked crystal methamphetamine get to the brain quickly, release a lot of dopamine, and are highly addictive. Drugs taken orally, such as Ritalin (methylphenidate), don't get there quickly and don't produce much euphoria. We talk about their positive effects at the end of this section.

2. When stimulants are abused, they can produce immediate health hazards.

Stimulants activate the heart, and they can produce a fatal cardiac arrhythmia. That's how people usually die from these drugs. No drugs do just one thing, and stimulants are typical in that regard. They do more than just increase the "addiction-promoting" chemical dopamine. They also increase a related chemical called norepinephrine, or noradrenaline. This neurochemical is responsible for much of the flight-or-fight response of the body. It makes your heart rate and blood pressure rise, raises your blood sugar, and generally prepares your body for emergency. Whenever you take cocaine or methamphetamine, you get the flight-or-fight response along with the pleasurable effects, your heart rate increases, and your blood pressure goes up. This can lead to heart attacks, strokes, hemorrhages, and other cardiovascular injury. There seems to be an equal chance (about 1 in 10,000) of a heart attack with each dose of drug. The risk is the same for the first use as for the hundredth. Repeated use of these drugs, however, can cause small strokes and brain damage.

3. The greatest risk of stimulant abuse is addiction and all its consequences.

Health hazards pale in comparison to the consequences of addiction. The problem is that once a person is addicted to a drug, the drug controls his life. Everything he does is directed to getting more of the drug. This compulsive behavior corrupts relationships, destroys financial security, and often leads to a loss of freedom in jail.

4. With repeated use of addictive drugs, the good feelings wear off, and the addict uses drugs just to stop feeling bad.

Because drugs repeatedly and strongly activate the pleasure centers of the brain, they change its response to "natural" stimuli, such as food and sex, to one that only wants drugs. This is the most ironic aspect of addiction—a person starts out trying to feel really good, but eventually cannot feel good with anything and just takes drugs to stop feeling bad. This is called anhedonia (inability to feel pleasure), and many addicts talk about it. Nothing tastes good, sex is uninteresting, only getting the drug and using it is important. We believe this occurs when the pleasure circuits in the reward system have experienced so much dopamine that they have become tolerant to it (see Chapter 2, Drug Basics). After so much stimulation, the brain "turns down" its sensitivity to dopamine. As a result, the addict is far less sensitive to the ordinary pleasures life provides. So nothing feels good.

5. Ritalin (methylphenidate) and other drugs for ADHD are safe stimulants when used as a doctor prescribes.

Ritalin (methylphenidate) and other drugs for ADHD are safe when used properly. These drugs are given orally and don't produce the euphoria of illegal stimulants. So long as a doctor monitors the person's health, he is quite safe. Because they are taken orally, they get into the brain slowly. They have to pass through the stomach, through the liver, and then into the bloodstream. They release dopamine, but so slowly that the addictive euphoric effects are not a problem. What they do stimulate is attention and focus.

Why do these drugs suppress hyperactivity? The easy answer is that we don't know, but we have some speculations. Some scientists believe that children with ADHD have a deficiency in the reward system, and this prevents them from paying attention to their work. It may also lead them to seek more novelty in their environments, so they become hyperactive in seeking more stimulation. When the ADHD drugs increase their levels of dopamine in the brain, they don't have to seek more of it through novelty, and they can pay attention better.

6. Diet stimulants and "natural" compounds with "Ephedra" should be treated with care.

Ephedrine and caffeine are sold as over-the-counter diet aids or "natural" Ritalin, but they probably should not be used by kids.

A huge number of preparations are available on the market. Ephedrine is viewed as safe and natural because it has been used in China for centuries to treat asthma. This is true when it is used in small doses, but too much ephedrine also revs up the cardiovascular system because it stimulates the flight-or-fight chemical norepinephrine. It doesn't get into the brain very well, and it doesn't raise dopamine, so it cannot bring about the increase in focus and attention of methylphenidate (Ritalin). It can make a person a little jittery, but it doesn't improve attention. The good news is that it is not addictive. However, it causes a rapid heart rate and elevated blood pressure. This effect makes people think they are getting a better workout, but they are just stimulating the heart artificially.

Ephedrine is also used in diet aids because it is supposed to "burn fat." What it does is release fat to use as an energy source. But without increased exercise to burn it off, the fat just goes back

143

to where it started. A lot of adolescents, especially girls, get into dieting and find these compounds attractive. *Our recommendation is that no child should take these stimulants for dieting.* They have not been tested for safety or effectiveness—we don't even know that they are safe for adults, much less children.

Finally, what do we say about the stimulant of choice in this culture—caffeine? Many people seem to think of it as a nutrient not a drug despite the fact that it is a mild stimulant. It does not work the same way that methylphenidate and amphetamine do, and we have little evidence that it is addictive. People's bodies adapt to it, so when you don't get your morning cup of coffee you can have a headache and feel a little down. The same thing happens when your children don't get their three diet sodas each day. Caffeine does stimulate the heart a little, but doesn't usually cause trouble unless someone has high blood pressure. Still, it is a drug, and we should teach our children to think about it (as we should think about it ourselves) whenever they put a chemical in their bodies.

TALKING WITH KIDS ABOUT STIMULANTS

• Teach kids that all stimulants are not the same. The fact that they or some of their friends take Ritalin or Adderal (a type of amphetamine) does not mean they are addicts. In fact, you can tell them that government studies show that kids taking Ritalin (methylphenidate) are at less risk of substance abuse than the population at large.

• If you need to have this conversation, explain that Ritalin and Adderal are very specially selected and tested by the government and drug companies to provide the stimulation of attention that people need without the side effects of euphoria and addiction.

• Kids shouldn't take Ritalin from a friend. Some kids think it can make their performance in school better. Explain that they should *never* take a medicine unless a doctor gives it to them.

• Explain that having ADHD is just a consequence of the way a person's brain developed, and sometimes it needs some help to pay attention properly. Drugs such as Ritalin provide that help, and they work well if they are used just as the doctor orders.

• Kids need to understand that although diet and exercise supplements such as ephedrine may make them feel stimulated, most of what they are getting is increased cardiovascular activity, and that's not good for them. This is not exercise in a pill. If they want cardiovascular stimulation they need to get out a do some serious exercise. They'll feel better and be thinner and stronger as well.

• Emphasize that they should never smoke or snort a stimulant. This is the fastest route to addiction, because the brain just loves a fast and strong rise in dopamine.

• Explain how stimulants tap into the most basic part of our brain to control our behavior. Talk about a favorite food they crave and point out that craving a drug is similar, only much, much more intense.

• Explain that addictions lead people to spend all their money on drugs, all of their time thinking about them, and possibly to spending a lot of time in jail.

• Explain tolerance to stimulants by using the example of a food your child eats so much that he becomes bored with it—pizza, chocolate cake, whatever. Hopefully, the child can see that too much of a good thing spoils it. Then make the connection to the pleasure centers of the brain. Drugs give them too much stimulation.

• Kids should know that they can die the first time they use these drugs. It's not likely, but it can happen.

• Even if they don't die, the repeated abuse of stimulants can damage the brain and heart. Stimulants raise blood pressure, and if they have a weak blood vessel, like a weak place in a balloon, it might blow out.

14. WHAT TO DO NOW?

Now that you've read this book, it's important to think about what to do with the information. There many possibilities. First of all, we recommend going back to Chapter 1, Communication Is Key, and reconsidering the ways in which you communicate with children about drugs, their bodies, and the choices that they make. With more information under your belt, you'll probably feel more confident about both raising and answering questions. Think about how to work your new information into conversations around the dinner table or during drives in the car. Remember that a talk about drugs doesn't have to be a long, emotionally or intellectually taxing event. A knowledgeable comment or thoughtful answer can go a long way, and now you are more prepared to offer them.

If you're a parent, consider becoming active with your new knowledge outside of your own family. Engage with leaders in your community, school, or religious groups to initiate discussions or programs that can begin a productive dialogue about drugs and drug-related issues with the children in your community. There are probably many people in your community (including yourself!) with valuable knowledge and experience that could be brought together to begin the process. Organizing a parents' forum at school could be a great contribution. You know what the important issues are, and you could help to make decisions about how to structure a workshop or panel discussion at your school, church, or community organization. Talk with a school counselor, science teacher, youth minister, or YMCA program director about putting a program together—you might be surprised by the enthusiasm you find.

Remember, you don't have to be an expert to be a valuable contributor to such a project. School systems (even the smallest ones) often have health educators who are always looking for effective ways to teach children about drugs and the process of making healthy decisions. You could be a valuable resource for them. Make an appointment to sit down and talk about what drug education strategies are in place in your school system, and see if those can be supplemented or improved.

If you're a teacher, think about how to incorporate the information in this book into your academic lessons—and this suggestion doesn't just apply to "science" teachers. Armed with the background on what drugs are predominant and how they work, we can imagine a language arts teacher incorporating literary works related to drug issues or a social studies teacher focusing on current approaches to the "war on drugs" and how those approaches are consistent or inconsistent with the scientific realities of drug effects or approaches to treatment. Physical education teachers and athletic coaches have great opportunities for influence as well. Questions related to performance-enhancing drugs and nutritional supplements could be answered as students are prepared for training regimens or health classes.

Whatever you do, do something. Don't let an opportunity to teach and guide your children pass you by. Remember what you learned earlier—the child's brain is a work in progress. Be part of it.

ADDITIONAL RESOURCES

Sources of information about drugs must be both reliable and up-to-date. In our experience, most sources do not meet these criteria. We have posted a list of what we believe are the most reliable and current sources on our website:

www.buzzed.org

You can also find helpful, up-to-date information in our books *Buzzed: The Straight Facts about the Most Used and Abused Drugs from Alcohol to Ecstasy* and *Pumped: Straight Facts for Athletes about Drugs, Supplements, and Training.*

Effiective school programs are being developed by Communities of Concern:

www.communitiesofconcern.org

INDEX

asthma medicine, 77, 132, 134, 143
athletics:
    "smokeless" tobacco and, 109–10,
       111, 113
    see also steroids
atropine, 35, 86
attention deficit disorder (ADD), 46
attention deficit hyperactivity disorder
    (ADHD), 108, 142–43, 145
authoritative vs. authoritarian parents, 18
automatic functions, 40

barbiturates, 61, 68, 115, 116
belladonna alkaloids, 86, 89
binge drinking, 20, 61, 66–68
    definition of, 59, 66–68
    reasons for, 67
bipolar disorder, 88
birth control pills, 34, 38
blood alcohol levels, 62–63, 64, 72, 73
blood pressure, 37–38, 78
bloodstream, drugs and, 36–37, 48
body, teaching care and respect for,
    15–16
body-building chemicals, 129
    see also steroids
body processes, drugs and, 35–38, 48
brain:
    alcohol and, 25, 41, 60, 64–66, 68,
       70–71, 74–75
    caffeine and, 33, 43, 77, 80–81, 83
    cocaine and, 43, 60, 139
    development of, 24–25, 64–66,
       74–75
    drugs and, 40–41, 48–49
    Ecstasy and, 121–24, 126–27
    excitatory vs. inhibitory influences
       on, 69
    GHB and, 127–28, 129
    hallucinogens and, 86, 89–90
    hormones and, 135
    ketamine and, 130
    marijuana and, 43, 96, 99–101, 104
    opiates and, 43, 114, 115, 116–17
    reward system of, 42–43, 46, 47,
       49, 60, 71, 136, 137–43, 145

stimulants and, 137–41
suppression-rebound-suppression
    pattern and, 68, 75
Buzzed (Kuhn, Swartzwelder, and
    Wilson), 53, 149

caffeine, 34, 47, 77–83, 144
    brain and, 33, 43, 77, 80–81, 83
    children's use of, 77, 78, 81–82
    discovery of, 35
    most important things to know
       about, 78–82
    as nonaddictive, 42
    parent's use of, 82–83
    physical effects of, 77–78, 80–81,
       82–83
    sources of, 33, 77, 78, 82
    talking with children about, 82–83
    varying levels of, 78–79
    withdrawal and, 39, 41, 42, 81
cardiac arrhythmia, 141
catabolic steroids, 132, 133
Central Intelligence Agency (CIA), 85,
    89
central nervous system, 127
    caffeine and, 77, 78
    see also brain
"chasing the high," 61
chewing tobacco, 106, 109–11, 113
children:
    brain development of, 24–25
    cigarettes as number one addiction
       concern for, 42
    fostering decision making by,
       19–20, 70
    importance of parent's listening to,
       17–18
    influence of media on, 17, 19
    information processing by, 16–17,
       19
    peer pressure and, 19–20, 44,
       45–46, 70
    privacy issues and, 27–28
    trust between parents and, 17, 19,
       27
    warning signs of drug use by, 26–30

monkeys, medicinal foods eaten by, 34
morphine, 34, 35, 114
Mothers Against Drunk Driving
 (MADD), 73, 74
motivation, 100–101, 105
"munchies," 98
mushrooms, psilocybin, 84, 85

narcotics, definition of, 34
National Center on Addiction and
 Substance Abuse, 21
National Institutes of Health, 98–99
National Survey on Drug Abuse, 67
neurons, 40
neurotoxins, 123–24
New York, N.Y., 36
nicotine, 24, 35, 47, 106–13
 addictiveness of, 41–42, 107–8,
  111–12
 ADHD and, 108
 brain's reward system and, 43
 forms of, 33, 106
 legal issues and, 54, 55–56
 most important things to know
  about, 107–11
 physical effects of, 106–7, 109–11,
  113
 reasons for use of, 107, 110–11
 "smokeless" tobacco and, 44, 106,
  109–11, 113
 talking with children about, 111–13
 see also cigarettes
nicotine gum and patches, 33, 106
"nightcaps," 63
nitrous oxide, 91, 92, 93
norepinephrine, 143
nose, drugs transmitted to bloodstream
 through, 36–37
nose drops, 37–38, 39, 40
nutritional supplements, 32, 34

opiates and sedatives, 34, 35, 76,
 114–19
 addictiveness of, 41–42, 115–16
 brain and, 43, 114, 115, 116–17
 in combination, 116–17

most important things to know
 about, 115–17
overdoses from, 114–15, 116,
 118–19
physical effects of, 117–18
range of, 114
talking with children about, 117–19
oral cancer, 110
over-the-counter medications, 33, 69
 as caffeine source, 77, 80

painkillers, 86
 see also opiates and sedatives
parents:
 authoritative vs. authoritarian, 18
 children's privacy and, 27–28
 consistency from, 20–21
 disclosure of previous drug experiences of, 23–24
 drug use by, 45, 47
 further options for, 147–48
 "hands-on" vs. "hands-off"
  approaches by, 21–22
 importance of listening by, 17–18
 as role models, 22–24, 57–58,
  75–76, 82–83
 sources of advice for, 21, 147–48
 as teachers to their children, 15–17
 trust between children and, 17, 19,
  27
"party" or "club" drugs, 120–30
 range of, 120
 see also specific drugs
PCP, 86, 89
peer pressure, 19–20, 44, 45–46, 70
performance-enhancing drugs, see
 steroids
plants, drugs derived from, 35
police departments, as information
 sources, 54–55, 73
"post-hallucinogen perceptual disorder," 88–89
prenatal brain development, 25
prescription medications, 33–34
privacy, rules on, 27–28
professional help, importance of, 46–47

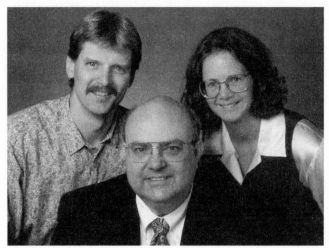

From left: Scott Swartzwelder, Wilkie Wilson, and Cynthia Kuhn.

About the Authors

Cynthia Kuhn is a professor of pharmacology at Duke University Medical Center and heads the Pharmacological Sciences Training Program at Duke. She is married with two teenaged children.

Scott Swartzwelder is a professor of psychology at Duke University and a clinical professor of psychiatry at Duke University Medical Center. He is also a research career scientist and has served as the program specialist in alcoholism and drug dependence for the Department of Veterans Affairs. He is married with three young children.

Wilkie Wilson is a professor of pharmacology at the Duke University Medical Center. He is also a research career scientist and has served as neurobiology program specialist for the Department of Veterans Affairs. He is married with two daughters.